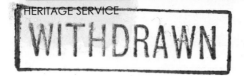

Understanding
Asthma

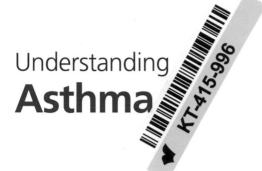

KT-415-996

Professor Jon Ayres

Published by Family Doctor Publications Limited
in association with the British Medical Association

© Family Doctor Publications 1997–2008
Updated 1999, 2000, 2001, 2002, 2003, 2005, 2006, 2008

Family Doctor Publications, PO Box 4664, Poole, Dorset BH15 1NN

ISBN-13: 978 1 903474 23 5
ISBN-10: 1 903474 23 X

Contents

About the author

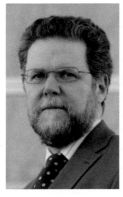

Professor Jon Ayres
After appointments as Professor of Respiratory Medicine and Professor of Environmental and Occupational Medicine in the University of Aberdeen, the author is now Professor of Environmental and Respiratory Medicine in the University of Birmingham. He has a special interest in asthma and the effects of outdoor and indoor air pollution on the lungs.
(Photo courtesy of Asthma UK.)

What is asthma?

The variability of asthma

Most people would recognise asthma in a child or adult as attacks of wheezy breathlessness, sometimes on exertion, sometimes at rest, sometimes mild, sometimes severe. Some would recognise specific 'triggers' – for example, animals, fumes, pollens. Some might think of asthma as a condition of children, some as a condition able to affect someone of any age. Some would regard it as an occasional nuisance requiring intermittent treatment only, others as a persistent, significant problem needing continuous treatment. Surely they can't all be right?

In a way they can, although it is this wide range of factors involved in asthma that makes it difficult to come up with a simple definition.

How can asthma be defined?

The word 'asthma' is used as a blanket term to cover a condition characterised by episodes of breathlessness caused by intermittent narrowing of the bronchial tubes – or airways – within the lung.

The respiratory system

The airways (trachea, bronchi and bronchioles) and airspaces within the lungs supply oxygen to and remove carbon dioxide from the body.

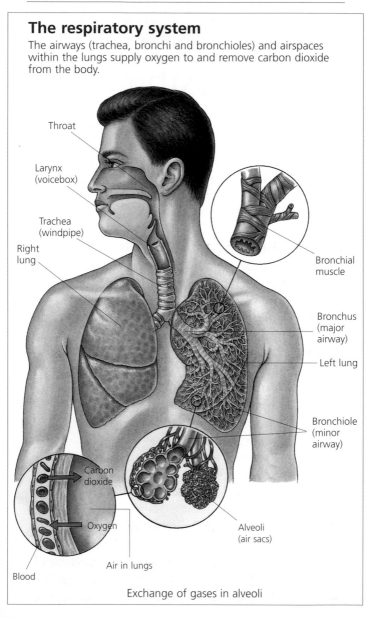

Throat

Larynx (voicebox)

Trachea (windpipe)

Right lung

Bronchial muscle

Bronchus (major airway)

Left lung

Bronchiole (minor airway)

Carbon dioxide

Oxygen

Alveoli (air sacs)

Blood

Air in lungs

Exchange of gases in alveoli

There are many factors that contribute to the development of asthma in the first instance and many that can induce attacks. In addition, these will vary from individual to individual.

The best definition is that asthma is a condition in which the airways within the lung are inflamed and so are more sensitive to specific factors (triggers) that cause the airways to narrow, reducing airflow through them and making the individual breathless and/or wheezy. This sensitivity of the airways enjoys the medical label 'bronchial hyper-reactivity'. In the surgery or clinic doctors use the term 'twitchy tubes'!

Normal breathing and asthma

So, why should this sensitivity result in the symptoms so well recognised by each individual with asthma? During most of our waking hours (and all those spent asleep) we are unaware of the gentle movement of the chest which allows oxygen-rich air to be inhaled and waste air, laden with carbon dioxide, to be expelled. We do this automatically because the natural tendency of the lungs and the chest wall is to collapse inwards, so automatic nerve pathways monitor the levels of oxygen and carbon dioxide in the blood and make the chest and therefore the lungs expand to open them up. This easy, untroubled breathing all depends upon air getting in and out of the lung through the branching system of bronchial tubes without any resistance.

Problems arise when the bronchial tubes narrow down, making the flow of air more difficult. In asthma, the narrowing occurs mostly in the smaller bronchial tubes, of which the smallest are about the diameter of a human hair, which open out into the alveoli (or air sacs). Each of these is about the size of the full stop at the end of this sentence, and this is where the inhaled oxygen diffuses easily into the blood vessels covering their surface and the carbon dioxide equally easily diffuses out.

If you spread all the alveoli in a pair of human lungs out, they would cover the area of a tennis court, which shows how well the lungs are suited to exchanging gases easily.

When the bronchial tubes narrow in asthma (the reasons for which I will explain), the flow of air through them drops quite quickly, so to overcome this resistance the chest wall muscles have to work harder to get the air in and out at the rate required to keep oxygen supplies constant. This becomes noticeable to that individual – he or she has to work harder to breathe and becomes breathless. As any musician knows, if you blow air through narrow tubes, noise will be generated – wheezing.

So asthma is not one disease: it covers a multitude of different patterns. Like the word 'cancer' it tells you roughly what sort of condition we are dealing with, what ballpark we are in. Under that general heading you will find a range of severities, a range of triggering factors and a range of outcomes. It logically follows that what is good for one person with asthma may be unsuitable for another.

Asthma is a very individual condition and management needs to be personalised because of the variety of factors that underlie each individual's asthma.

The mechanics of breathing

To inhale air, muscles in the chest wall contract, lifting the ribs and pulling them outwards. The diaphragm moves downward enlarging the chest cavity further. Reduced air pressure in the lungs causes air to enter the lungs from outside. Breathing out reverses this.

Breathing in (inhalation)

Air in

Chest muscles contract lifting ribs

Diaphragm descends

Breathing out (exhalation)

Air out

Chest muscles relax

Diaphragm ascends

Nasal passages

Mouth

Trachea (windpipe)

Lungs

Lung volume increases

Diaphragm

Lung volume decreases

KEY POINTS

■ Asthma is not one disease. Like the word 'cancer' it covers a multitude of different patterns

■ As a result of the wide range of factors involved in causing asthma and the variety of responses that the body's airways make, it is not easy to define asthma simply

How much asthma is there?

Is asthma increasing?

Between the 1970s and the 1990s asthma increased in the number of people with a diagnosis and the number of attacks that they were having. For instance, over that period there was around a fivefold increase in the numbers of patients presenting to their GP with an attack of asthma, more so in children but to some extent in adults. There was also an increase in hospital admissions up to the early 1990s, again particularly in children, possibly reflecting the fact that parents are more likely to seek medical advice for their children than for themselves, although other factors are also likely to play a part.

Since that time the increase has been much slower, but there has been no real evidence of a substantial fall in numbers affected. Gratifyingly, the rise stopped in the early 1990s and is now declining, although some markers of asthma remain high.

Asthma is the most common condition to be found in western populations, affecting over five million individuals in England and Wales alone. In children, boys are more likely to be affected than girls, while in adult life the condition is slightly more common in women.

Why did asthma increase?

It is possible that some of the increase mentioned above is a result of doctors now using the word 'asthma', whereas before they would have used 'wheezy bronchitis', but this cannot explain the greater part of the rise. Exposure to allergens in the home, viral infections, and aspects of the indoor environment such as central heating, air pollution, the stress of modern living – even the treatments used for asthma itself – have all been blamed for the increase, but there is limited evidence to support these ideas.

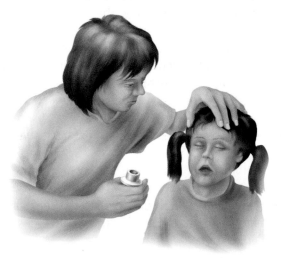

More recently it has been suggested that the increase in asthma is related to a reduction in infections – in other words, the more germs there are the less asthma is likely to occur. This has been dubbed the 'hygiene hypothesis', the basic idea being that with our hygienic modern lifestyle our immune systems, having less need to respond to infection, respond to allergens thus leading to asthma. It has also been suggested that the various germs that live in our intestines may also play a role in determining whether we develop asthma.

Deaths from asthma

Fortunately, death from asthma is not common. In the mid-1960s a short-lived epidemic of deaths caused by asthma occurred, which some thought might be the result of a toxic effect of one of the asthma inhalers on sale at the time. This has been disputed over the years and other factors may have been of importance; it is unlikely that we shall ever know the complete story surrounding that event.

In fact, most asthma deaths are caused by undertreatment of patients and it has been shown that two-thirds of asthma deaths would have been preventable with adequate treatment.

Between the 1970s and the 1990s, there was a further slight rise in asthma deaths in patients over the age of 50, although this, again, settled down in the 1990s. Why this has occurred is not clear, although in the older patient differentiating between asthma and chronic bronchitis is often difficult and this may have led to a change in diagnostic fashion.

Geographical differences

There are certainly some parts of the UK where asthma admissions and GP attendances are more common, and other areas where they are less so. However, the differences are modest and do not form a clear-cut geographical pattern, unlike attacks of acute bronchitis, which are higher in the north, becoming less so towards the south.

Although the differences within the UK are slight, there are quite huge differences in the distribution of asthma in different parts of the world. It is almost unheard of in Eskimos and black Africans living in rural areas, whereas in the Western Caroline Islands in the north Pacific Ocean, nearly 50 per cent of the inhabitants have asthma, with three-quarters of all children being affected.

Between these extremes are the westernised populations, such as people in the UK, Australia, New Zealand and other European countries, which all have roughly the same amount of asthma. Interestingly, those parts of the world with less asthma are those that are less encouraging to the survival of the house dust mite but where infections and parasitic infestations abound – further evidence to support the hygiene hypothesis.

KEY POINTS

- Over five million individuals in England and Wales alone have asthma

- Boys are more frequently affected than girls, but the condition is slightly more common in women than in men

Causes and triggers of asthma

Is asthma hereditary?

Most people know that asthma can 'run in families' and there is undoubtedly a hereditary component to this condition, particularly in allergic asthma. The genetic factor is much less marked in patients where allergy is not involved.

An allergic reaction is an over-reaction of the immune defence system, in which it responds inappropriately to a normally harmless environmental substance, causing troublesome or even life-threatening effects.

How does asthma start?

The tendency to develop asthma is not absolute: it is not inherited in the way that eye colour and blood group are, and a patient with very severe asthma can have children who never develop the condition.

The role of environmental factors (for example, allergens, diet, exposure to passive smoking) is therefore paramount in the development – and exacerbation – of asthma. Nevertheless, it is clear that, in order for the 'seed' of asthma to germinate, the 'soil' must be right!

There is increasing evidence that the conditions for asthma can be prepared while the fetus is in the uterus and this may be affected by factors such as maternal smoking and even maternal diet during pregnancy when vitamin E seems to be important. Critically however, factors acting during the first year or two of life may be the most important.

House dust mite and other factors

Against this background, many factors seem to be responsible for the first appearance of the symptoms of asthma. For instance, asthma beginning in adult life often seems to start following a 'cold' or viral

House dust mite

The house dust mite, shown here on the woven threads of a textile, is smaller than a full stop on this page. Dust mites live in carpets, mattresses and other soft furnishings. Their dead bodies and faeces can trigger asthma.

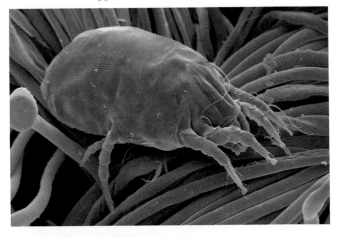

infection; exposure to a substance in the workplace is a common and often under-recognised cause of asthma (see page 87).

An important factor that can cause asthma, particularly in children, is an allergen (substance that induces an allergy) from the house dust mite. This little beast, smaller than a pin point, lives in our carpets, mattresses and furry toys. There can be as many as two million in each mattress!

When a susceptible individual is exposed to a protein in the faecal pellet of the mite over a period of time, the body's white cells become sensitive to this 'foreign substance'. As the protein is inhaled, a reaction to it occurs in the lining of the bronchial tubes, resulting in inflammation of the airways. The inflammation makes the lining irritable so that any further exposure, to either the house dust mite or any other potential trigger factor, will result in narrowing of the bronchial tubes and the symptoms of asthma. There are other things that may be contributory factors to the initiation of asthma. Smoking by the mother during pregnancy and exposure to passive cigarette smoke in

Factors contributing to the development of asthma

- Inheritance (genetic factors)
- Mother smoking during pregnancy
- Passive smoking in childhood
- Allergens (especially house dust mite)
- Infections
- Occupational exposures, e.g. chemicals

The airways of the lungs

The bronchi in our lungs are made up of rings of smooth muscle. The airway is coated with mucus that sticks to inhaled contaminants and lined with cilia cells which waft the mucus out of the lungs.

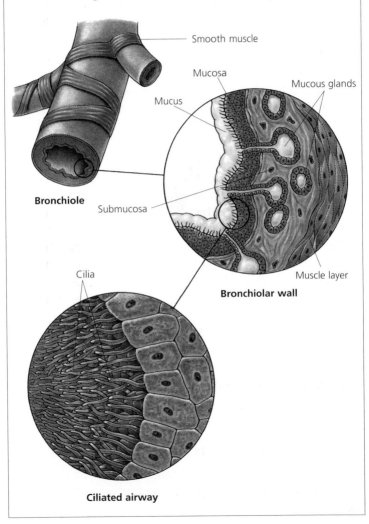

Smooth muscle

Mucosa

Mucous glands

Mucus

Bronchiole

Submucosa

Muscle layer

Bronchiolar wall

Cilia

Ciliated airway

childhood may contribute in some cases and there is increasing evidence that diet may also play a role.

What happens during an asthma attack?
Airway inflammation

Asthma, then, is the result of inflammation, which makes the airways more irritable. Inflammation is the body's response to a range of assaults and is seen in many illnesses such as arthritis, colitis and dermatitis. Problems arise for the patient when the inflammation does not resolve and becomes long standing (or chronic), as is the case in asthma.

The normal airway is lined with a delicate protective layer called the mucosa or epithelium. This layer consists of various types of cell with different jobs. Some can produce mucus, whereas others help to clear the mucus from the airway by wafting the secretions up the bronchial tubes via movement of tiny fingers or cilia, which are found on the surface of these cells. These cilia are some of the first structures to be destroyed by cigarette smoke, which also stimulates increased mucus production because the smoke causes inflammation. This is the reason why smokers cough up phlegm – the cilia no longer work. In some patients with asthma, cough is also important and this is hardly surprising now that we have seen that asthma is an inflammatory and irritant condition.

Below the epithelium, a second layer (the submucosa) lies over a spiral sheet of muscle which, in asthma, contracts when a patient inhales a trigger such as grass pollen.

There are three separate processes that lead to airway narrowing and wheezy breathlessness:

How asthma affects the airways

During an asthma attack, the muscle walls of the airways contract, causing their internal diameter to narrow. Increased mucus secretion and inflammation of the airways' inner linings cause further narrowing.

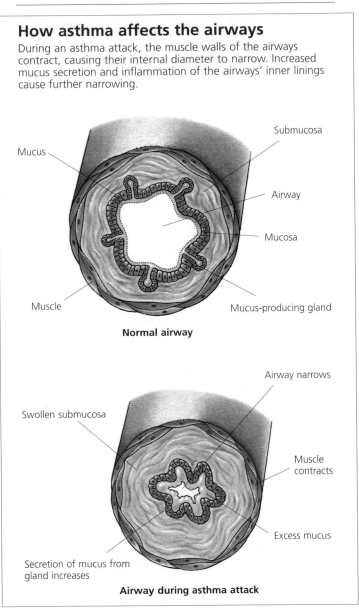

Normal airway

Submucosa

Mucus

Airway

Mucosa

Muscle

Mucus-producing gland

Airway during asthma attack

Airway narrows

Swollen submucosa

Muscle contracts

Excess mucus

Secretion of mucus from gland increases

1 First, the middle layer of the airway (the submucosa) becomes swollen.

2 Second, the mucous glands produce more secretions (which have to be coughed up to clear the airways).

3 Third, the smooth muscle contracts as a result of release of substances from inflammatory cells.

As asthma becomes persistent, scar tissue is laid down in the submucosa, causing a degree of irreversible airway narrowing. This has been labelled 'airway remodelling' and, although the extent varies from individual to individual, this appears to be a fundamental part of chronic asthma.

The net result of these three effects is to narrow the airways, so different forms of treatment have been devised to attack each of these three components.

In asthma, symptoms can occur for no obvious reason or may be caused by a clear-cut exposure to a known 'trigger factor' such as grass pollen during the summer. Equally, the airway narrowing can reverse with improvement of symptoms, either spontaneously or after the use of a reliever drug. It is this variability that is so characteristic of asthma. We take advantage of this both when making the diagnosis and when devising ways of keeping asthma under control.

Main trigger factors in asthma

In a susceptible person, any of the following triggers can start an asthma attack. An individual soon recognises which factors affect him or her.

Exercise

This is a particularly obvious trigger in children, where it may often be the only thing that brings out asthmatic symptoms. The problem is that breathlessness on exertion is often attributed to non-fitness rather than asthma. The schoolboy is then felt to be not fit enough to play as a forward on the football field (putting us in danger of producing a nation of asthmatic goalkeepers!).

Allergens

Grass pollen is the most frequently recognised allergic trigger but animals, particularly cats and horses, are potent causes of asthma attacks. This occurs because exposure to the allergen releases the allergy antibody, IgE, which sets in train a series of events making inflammation of the airways – and hence asthma symptoms – worse. Chronic exposure to allergens may result in more persistent symptoms, and the importance of animals in the house may be missed as the patient claims to be able to stroke the cat without 'getting an attack', not realising that long-term exposure is causing chronic symptoms.

Fumes, dusts and odours

Cigarette smoke is a potent trigger for many patients, as are dusty environments, where the dust acts as an irritant. Odours, such as scent or aftershave, can be a trigger for certain individuals but this is not an allergy. Presumably, it is an irritant reaction to the chemicals involved, and the best treatment is avoidance where possible, although this may have important consequences.

'Colds' and viruses

Viral infections (such as the common cold) are the most common trigger for asthma across the age spectrum. Antibiotics are effective in treating only bacterial infections, which occur rarely in asthma; viruses are completely unaffected by antibiotics, which have little or no place in the management of asthma but are consistently yet inappropriately prescribed for episodes of worsening asthma.

Emotions and stress

Children often become more wheezy at birthday parties, where the combination of excitement and exertion makes asthma more obvious. Asthma was for years regarded as a neurotic condition, but it is now clear that emotional factors act as triggers, not initiators, of asthma, and may consistently increase the twitchiness of the airways, making the attack more likely. Excitement, grief and stress can all trigger an attack.

We have occasionally found patients to have attacks when attending funerals and in other such stressful situations.

Climate and pollution

Many patients with asthma know that their condition is affected by the weather, but there is no uniform pattern. Some prefer cold to warm weather; others prefer hot, dry atmospheres. You, the patient, know best and will usually adjust your behaviour and treatment accordingly.

Air pollution episodes can cause exacerbations of asthma, more in those with severe asthma, ozone being the main cause during the summer and particles in the winter.

There is, however, no direct evidence that exposure to air pollution at current levels will turn a non-asthmatic person into someone with asthma.

Cold air, foods and occupational triggers

These can all trigger asthma in susceptible individuals.

Illustrative case histories
Case history 1: childhood asthma

John is seven years old and his mother, who had hay fever when younger, had noticed that he had begun to cough when running around in the garden. She had taken him to the GP who had prescribed antibiotics with no benefit on three separate occasions.

The symptoms became more persistent and it was only when he developed wheeze on exertion during a games lesson at school that the penny dropped, and a diagnosis of asthma was made. John was prescribed a bronchodilator (tube-opening) inhaler to be used when

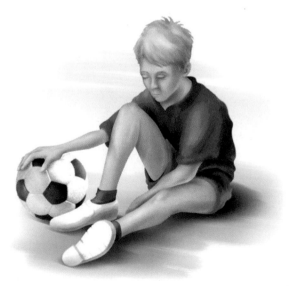

Sometimes asthma is diagnosed only when a child develops wheeze during a games lesson.

he has symptoms, since which time he has been well and able to play without getting breathless.

Case history 2: fur allergy

Caroline, a 27-year-old woman with long-standing asthma, was referred to a chest physician because of worsening symptoms over the previous two months. She was known to have many allergic triggers for her asthma, including grass and tree pollens and a number of furry animals.

As part of the assessment, the doctor visited her at home to be greeted by 14 cats which, it emerged, she bred and showed, a fact of which her GP was unaware.

Caroline had an extremely strong skin test reaction to cat fur but fervently denied that stroking the cats made her worse. It was clear that the cats were a major cause of her continuing asthma, providing a constant exposure to allergen, which effectively gave

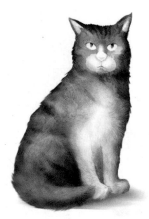

Asthma can worsen as a result of exposure to animal fur.

her recurrent, virtually continuous, asthma episodes. She would not get rid of the cats, her best friends, and a balance has had to be struck between bad asthma caused by exposure to allergens and the benefits of keeping her friends and companions.

Case history 3: air pollution

David, a man in his 20s with severe asthma, had had some difficulty in controlling his asthma during the previous autumn. He had increased his inhalers and his GP had given him two courses of steroid tablets. Coming up to Christmas, his asthma at last seemed to be stabilising somewhat, when a five-day air pollution episode hit Birmingham, reaching peak levels on Christmas Eve. By that day David's asthma had become very much worse and, in spite of more steroid tablets and increasing use of his nebuliser, he had to be admitted to hospital – a most unacceptable way to spend Christmas!

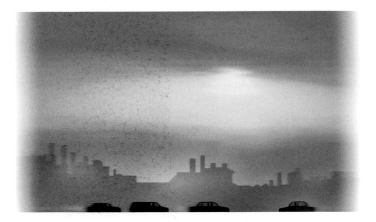

Air pollution episodes can cause exacerbations of asthma.

Case history 4: pollen sensitivity

In June 1994, a severe thunderstorm struck southern Britain, moving from the Southampton area, up through London and then northwards through East Anglia. During this period, hundreds of patients presented to accident and emergency departments with asthma attacks. Many had no idea that they were asthmatic, although most admitted to wheezing from hay fever (that is, they had had asthma but had not realised).

We now know that the combination of the cold front associated with thunderstorms and the rising humidity before the storm (causing rupture of the pollen grains and release of large amounts of grass pollen allergen into the air) act together, in these circumstances, to produce what are effectively acute allergic asthma attacks.

Case history 5: perfume sensitivity

Georgina had worked for 22 years in the cosmetic department of the local department store. After a viral infection one autumn, she developed asthma which initially proved easy to treat by the usual means.

However, over a year she developed worsening symptoms, particularly cough, and the main trigger appeared to be scents. She stopped using perfumes herself but, after an initial slight improvement, her symptoms clearly began to relate to her exposure to perfumes at the store. Eventually she had to give up her job (she was 58) and her symptoms improved immeasurably.

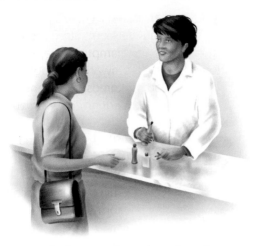

Perfume can be a trigger for asthma.

Interacting trigger factors

In many cases, two or more of these trigger factors will interact, and different combinations will be important for different individuals. Asthma is a very personal condition – what is good for one may not necessarily be good for another, and patterns of avoidance, treatment and planning in advance need to be organised for each individual.

KEY POINTS

■ Asthma can run in families, but a patient with quite severe asthma can have children who never develop the condition

■ The most important factor in initiating asthma, particularly in children, is the house dust mite

■ Symptoms may occur for no obvious reason, or may be caused by exposure to one or more trigger factors, such as exercise, viral infection, fumes and dusts, grief and stress, climate and pollution

■ Different combinations of trigger factors are important for different patients

Symptoms and diagnosis

Diagnosis of asthma is often difficult as the symptoms can easily be confused with other respiratory complaints. A firm diagnosis may be made after taking a history and undertaking tests.

What are the symptoms?

Asthma can present with one or more of four main symptoms:

- wheeze
- breathlessness
- cough
- chest tightness.

Wheeze and breathlessness are the most well recognised, usually coming on intermittently either in response to a recognised trigger or out of the blue. However, breathlessness without wheeze can frequently occur.

One symptom often not recognised as being caused by asthma is cough – either a dry cough or cough with phlegm – which typically occurs at night or on exercise. Failure to recognise that cough can be caused by asthma often results in a diagnosis of bronchitis being made. Attacks of bronchitis are usually treated by antibiotics, which is quite an inappropriate treatment for asthma. More than two episodes of persistent cough – with or without wheeze or breathlessness – should raise the question of underlying asthma in the minds of both the patient and the doctor.

Four main symptoms of asthma

Wheeze and breathlessness, asthma's most common symptoms, may occur together or separately. Persistent cough is less well recognised and chest tightness may be apparent only on exertion.

- **Wheeze**
  With or without breathlessness, wheeze may occur in response to a trigger or for no obvious reason.

- **Breathlessness**
  Often associated with wheeze and cough, but may also occur alone.

- **Cough**
  Either a phlegm-producing or a dry cough may be a sign of asthma.

- **Chest tightness**
  Although often a symptom of asthma, chest tightness may be mistaken for a heart problem in older people.

  Waking at night because of asthma symptoms means poor control.

The fourth main symptom of asthma is chest tightness. Often, this occurs on exertion and, when this happens in an older patient, a diagnosis of angina may be made, and it may be quite a difficult problem for the doctor to sort out.

Although the symptoms of asthma often occur for no apparent reason, characteristically they can wake patients and are often a problem on waking in the morning. Waking at night with asthma means that the asthma is being inadequately treated.

How is asthma diagnosed?

The trouble with these symptoms is that they occur in many other types of lung – or heart – condition. So, a careful history of what the symptoms are, what sets them off, how long they last, how bad they are and whether there are any recognisable patterns of symptoms is essential to the doctor in helping him or her arrive at a diagnosis.

Although listening to the chest is part of any examination, very often in asthma it doesn't help the doctor a great deal. The absence of wheezing does NOT mean that asthma isn't the diagnosis!

Conversely, all that wheezes is not asthma – making the diagnosis of asthma quite difficult at times.

Breathing tests

Although a diagnosis of asthma may have been made on history alone, some simple tests are often used to help. In older patients, in whom heart complaints are common, an electrocardiogram (ECG or heart trace) may help, but breathing tests form the mainstay of the investigation of asthma.

Conditions that share the symptoms of asthma

The symptoms of asthma occur in some other respiratory disorders and a few heart conditions. This table shows in which diseases and how commonly the symptoms are seen.

Diagnosis	Wheeze	Breath-lessness	Cough	Chest tightness
Asthma	● ● ●	● ● ● ●	● ● ●	● ● ●
Chronic bronchitis	● ● ●	● ● ●	● ● ●	● ●
Emphysema	● ●	● ● ●	●	● ● ●
Bronchiectasis	● ●	● ●	● ● ● ●	● ●
Angina	●	● ●	●	● ● ● ●
Heart failure	● ●	● ● ● ●	● ●	● ●

● , Symptom not usually seen.   ● ● ● , Symptom often seen.

● ● , Symptom can be seen.   ● ● ● ● , Symptom virtually always seen.

There are two main types of breathing tests used in diagnosing asthma – peak-flow tests and spirometry. Both measure how narrow the airways may be because, the narrower the airways, the slower the flow of air through the tubes and the lower the readings.

The peak-flow meter
The peak-flow meter is small, cheap and robust, and gives an idea of the narrowness of the airways by measuring the maximum, or peak, rate at which air can be expelled. This is the method most likely to be used by GPs as a single reading in the surgery. However, you may be asked to use one to measure

Peak-flow meter

You may be asked to measure your peak flow several times each day using a peak-flow meter.

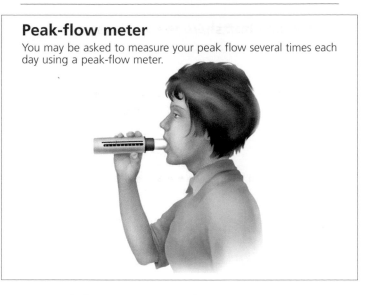

your peak flow two, three or four times a day to show variation in values over the day. A normal individual will show very little variation in peak flow over days and weeks, whereas the patient with asthma shows either consistent or intermittent variation.

A common pattern is the 'morning dip', values being lowest on waking. Sometimes the fall in peak flow is intermittent, often in response to a recognised trigger such as cat fur. Measuring peak flow in this way is particularly helpful if you complain of only intermittent symptoms.

Daily peak-flow self-monitoring can be extremely helpful in management plans by acting as an 'early warning system' to anticipate worsening asthma.

Spirometry

This is mostly used at chest clinics and in hospitals, although an increasing number of general practices

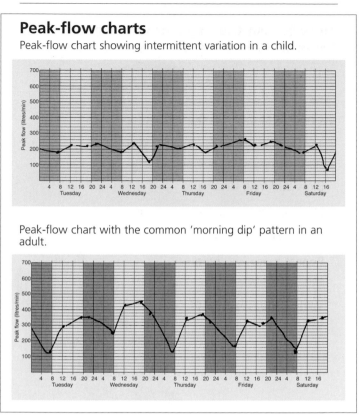

Peak-flow charts

Peak-flow chart showing intermittent variation in a child.

Peak-flow chart with the common 'morning dip' pattern in an adult.

now use spirometry. It measures not only how fast air can be blown out but also the amount blown out with each breath. Spirometry provides more information than peak flow and small spirometers for use at home are now becoming more available in some specialist chest clinics.

'Reversibility' tests

Sometimes these breathing tests are performed before and after inhalation of a bronchodilator drug, which

How to use the peak-flow meter

Your doctor or asthma nurse will show you how to use your peak-flow meter correctly. These instructions are a reminder.

1 Stand up if possible.

2 Check that cursor is on zero.

3 Take a deep breath in and place peak-flow meter in the mouth (hold horizontally), and close lips.

4 Blow suddenly and hard.

5 Note number indicated by cursor.

6 Return cursor to zero.

7 Repeat twice and obtain three readings.

8 Write down the best of the three readings.

Cursor

Scale

Mouthpiece

If in doubt always seek professional advice

opens the tubes. If the readings increase by 15 per cent or more after inhaling the drug, the airway narrowing is said to be reversible and confirms a diagnosis of asthma. Even patients with asthma do not always show reversibility on every occasion tested, but it is nevertheless a useful diagnostic test in patients in whom asthma is suspected.

Other breathing tests

If your diagnosis is difficult to sort out, you may be sent to a lung function laboratory; here more complicated tests are arranged, usually at the request of a hospital doctor.

KEY POINTS

- The four main symptoms of asthma are wheeze, breathlessness, cough and chest tightness

- Waking at night with asthma means that the asthma is being inadequately treated

- More than two episodes of persistent cough should suggest asthma

- Wheezing does not necessarily indicate asthma, and asthma does not necessarily involve wheezing

- Breathing tests are often used to help confirm the diagnosis

Prevention and self-help

Although a diagnosis of asthma may seem to lead inevitably to the use of drugs to control the condition, there are several ways in which you and your family can help reduce symptoms. Equally, there are some environmental modifications that are not believed to be of help.

Avoiding allergens

Although there is a degree of controversy about whether controlling allergen exposure in the home may improve asthma, on balance, at present, in someone with allergic asthma, the introduction of control systems is worth considering in some patients, although the measures can be expensive. With regard to controlling house dust mite (see page 13), the use of occlusive bedding is effective but extremely costly, unless simple polythene sheeting is used to enclose the mattress and each pillow completely. This makes for a very crinkly and sweaty bed, however! Sprays to kill the mites are ineffective on their own in controlling asthma. In theory, carpets and loose fittings should be removed and some recommend blinds instead of curtains. Cuddly toys should be put in the freezer for 12 hours a week to kill the mites. As these measures are time-consuming or expensive, inhaled therapy is a much easier method of controlling symptoms for most people.

Pets

Getting rid of domestic pets is a contentious issue. Where there is undoubted allergy to cats, dogs or rabbits, a balance has to be struck between control of asthma using inhalers and the grief that can be caused by banishing the pet! Nevertheless, long-term exposure to pets, even those that do not induce an obvious attack, can chronically worsen asthma by exposing a sensitised patient to high levels of allergen. In the person with more severe asthma, where control is more difficult,

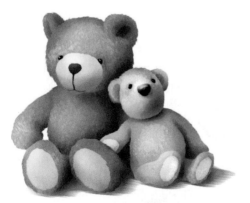

For children with asthma, cuddly toys should be put in the freezer for 12 hours every week to kill mites.

sometimes we have to insist on removal, although the results are not always as beneficial as we might wish.

I believe that patients' wishes are very important. Some would rather get rid of a pet than use inhalers; others would rather suffer asthma than lose what is often their best friend.

Only when beliefs and wishes cause risk to the patient should we be emphatic about parting with the pet.

Central heating
There is no direct evidence one way or the other that any particular form of central heating is either good or bad for patients with asthma. The belief that gas-fired central heating dries the air too much has been reported by some patients with asthma, but it is unlikely that this is a major problem. On the other hand, there are good theoretical reasons to believe that ducted or warm

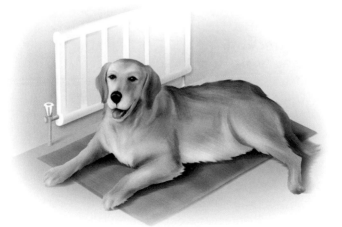

Both central heating and pets may be triggers for asthma.

air central heating may cause a problem, especially in those patients with allergy to house dust mite.

Unfortunately, it is extremely expensive to replace such systems, especially when there is no guarantee that the patient will improve after removal. I do, however, advise my patients to avoid installing these systems if they are putting in a new one.

Bedroom temperature

A famous doctor of the seventeenth century, Sir John Floyer, who himself had asthma, believed that when asthma woke a patient up at night this was due to 'the heat of the bed'! Equally, it has been said that sleeping with the bedroom window open, or at least keeping the air cool at night, is a help to people with asthma. In truth, there is no clear-cut answer. Some prefer the cooler night air; others will find that it causes them to wheeze more, particularly if they have to get up at night for some other reason. Again, it is up to you to adjust your environment according to what suits you best.

Viral infections

Viruses are an unavoidable cause of worsening asthma, but it makes sense to put off a visit to or from someone with a streaming cold! For mums and schoolchildren, however, this is unavoidable – children have to go to school and should not be kept off just because of the risk of catching a cold.

Food allergies

A small proportion of patients with asthma, particularly children, undoubtedly have food sensitivities. Again, a balance has to be struck between the wishes of the patient and the control of asthma.

True food allergy is not particularly common but is undoubtedly more common than many doctors believe. The diagnosis is often difficult and involves time-consuming tests. Skin tests can be very misleading and should not be relied on to diagnose or exclude food allergy. In an important minority, identifying a food or foods that worsen an individual's asthma can have a dramatic effect (see the Family Doctor Book *Understanding Allergies.*)

A clear history of, for example, wheezing within minutes of eating a peanut is easy to recognise, and the best treatment is avoidance. On the other hand, sensitivity to dairy products or wheat is more difficult to recognise because the effects are more chronic (long lasting) and not so dramatic.

Case history 1: nut allergy

Nick had had asthma since childhood and he had always known that peanuts made him worse and could cause very severe attacks. He had managed to prevent this by scrupulously avoiding all peanut-containing foods, often a difficult job! During his teens his asthma improved considerably but he still avoided peanuts. On the odd occasion when he took in a mouthful of food containing peanuts, he would immediately notice a tingling sensation in his mouth and would spit out the uneaten food. This usually prevented an attack.

One day, while eating a meal at the house of his new girlfriend, he suddenly realised that he had swallowed a mouthful of peanut-containing food. Within minutes, his tongue and lips had swollen and he had begun a severe asthma attack.

By the time he reached hospital he was blue and unconscious. Luckily, he had been taken there extremely quickly but he still required ventilation for a short period before recovering. His girlfriend and her mother were mortified as they had been unaware of his peanut allergy – one of the food allergies that patients rarely if ever grow out of – thus highlighting the dangers of 'hidden' food allergens.

If you think that you are sensitive to certain foods, you should be investigated by a doctor with relevant expertise.

Case history 2: wheat allergy

Carolyn was 35 years old and had had asthma since her teens. Initially, it had affected her quality of life, but she had managed to develop a career and generally had her asthma under good control. Over a period of two to three years, however, she began to suffer worsening symptoms and found that she was needing frequent courses of oral steroids. Concerned, she asked to be referred to hospital where drug treatment was increased to a maximum without success. She was then admitted to hospital to undergo a food exclusion regimen, which suggested that she might be sensitive to wheat products. When challenged with wheat in capsule form after a period of abstention, her asthma deteriorated over a week, confirming the suspicion. Since avoiding wheat, her asthma has been well controlled, although she is still on inhalers at moderate dose but she has only rarely needed a course of oral steroids.

If you are shown to have a problem, avoiding the foods is the only way forward. For foods that are not often eaten (for example, shellfish) avoidance is relatively straightforward. However, if you are sensitive to dairy products or wheat – two of the more commonly recognised problem foodstuffs – the diet may become particularly tiresome and antisocial, especially if your asthma symptoms are modest. Some patients would rather stick to a diet than take any drugs at all. Only rarely will asthma symptoms be completely controlled by dietary means, which should be seen as complementary to adequate medical treatment.

Cigarette smoke

Cigarette smoke is bad for asthma. Sadly, 15 to 20 per cent of patients with asthma smoke, and these patients are more likely to end up in hospital with acute asthma and to develop irreversible narrowing of their airways. If you smoke, you must try to stop by whatever means you can – this requires a great deal of help from relatives and friends. 'Just the one' *will* hurt, and offering you a cigarette is a far from friendly act.

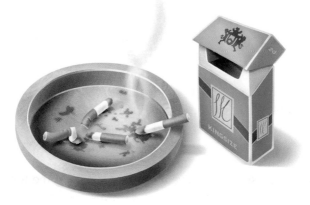

Cigarette smoke is bad for asthma.

Smoking cessation clinics are able to provide specific aid such as nicotine patches or new drugs that can aid smoking cessation, such as Zyban (bupropion) or Champix (varencline), which reduces the urge to smoke.

Inhaling other people's second-hand smoke (passive smoking) causes considerable suffering to children with asthma. The children of parents who smoke are more likely to have wheezy episodes and time off school than are children with non-smoking parents. This is most marked when both parents smoke, but maternal smoking seems to be more of a problem than that of the father, because children usually spend more time with their mums. The recent bans on smoking in public places has increased the risk of children being exposed to more cigarette smoke at home. It is now clear that passive cigarette smoke is even more toxic than previously thought, so every effort to reduce exposure should be taken.

Smoking during pregnancy increases the risk of the child being born with asthma, even allowing for all other risk factors such as family history.

Games and school

Exercise-induced asthma is common in children and can cause problems, with teachers accusing kids of 'not trying' or attempting to avoid games lessons, and their own school mates teasing them for 'being useless' and other colourful taunts. Sensible preparation can help. It is always a good idea for a child with asthma to take a relief inhaler (see page 47) about 15 minutes before going out to play games. If it is used just as he runs on to

Helping yourself or your child

- Don't smoke cigarettes

- Avoid 'colds' where possible

- Control allergen exposures

- Establish a self-management plan with the help of your doctor

- Keep teachers informed about your child's asthma and the need for access to inhalers on demand

- Where obvious triggers are known, avoid them

the pitch, symptoms will develop before the inhaler has a chance to work.

In some children, after the first episode of wheezing with exercise, there often follows a period when they can run long and hard without problems, which may last for the rest of the session. This so-called 'refractory period' sometimes, unfortunately, has the effect of reinforcing to a sceptical teacher or schoolmate that the child was always trying to 'skive'!

This brings up the whole subject of asthma in school. Many teachers are poorly informed about asthma, although it must be said that they are often very keen to know more if offered the chance. If you have a child with asthma, you should take the opportunity to tell your child's teachers about the need for your son or daughter to have ready access to a relief inhaler. All too often we hear of inhalers being locked away in the school secretary's office, which may be some distance from the school playing field. By explaining to the teachers how to allow the use of a relief inhaler without permitting its abuse, the teachers' worries about the perceived dangers of inhalers will be dispelled.

Sports and athletics

Many top sportsmen and sportswomen (such as Ian Botham and Paula Radcliffe) have asthma and are able to compete at the highest level. Some of the self-help advice given above for children is applicable to adults, particularly as far as use of inhalers before exertion is concerned. A warm-up period may help to some extent with the problems of exercise-induced symptoms when doing the first exercise of the day.

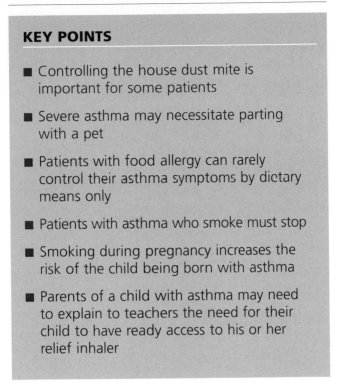

KEY POINTS

■ Controlling the house dust mite is important for some patients

■ Severe asthma may necessitate parting with a pet

■ Patients with food allergy can rarely control their asthma symptoms by dictary means only

■ Patients with asthma who smoke must stop

■ Smoking during pregnancy increases the risk of the child being born with asthma

■ Parents of a child with asthma may need to explain to teachers the need for their child to have ready access to his or her relief inhaler

Drugs used in the treatment of asthma

The three groups of drugs

The drugs used for the treatment of asthma can be divided into three main groups. These are known as:

- relievers
- preventers
- emergency (or reserve) drugs.

Relievers (bronchodilators)

These drugs act by relaxing the muscle in the walls of the airways, allowing the airway to open up and air to get in and out more easily. The result is that breathing is eased. These are also called bronchodilator drugs and are given in inhaled form, the inhaler usually being blue or sometimes green or grey in colour. Inhalers come in a range of different types.

In most cases, relief inhalers should be used when symptoms occur rather than on a regular basis, although, if you have more severe asthma, regular use may be needed on the advice of your doctor.

Preventers

These drugs act by reducing the inflammation in the airways, thus calming their irritability. In contrast to reliever inhalers, they must be taken on a regular basis, usually twice a day. In a way, they are like a toothbrush – regular use will keep you out of trouble! Indeed, many patients keep their preventer inhaler next to their toothbrush as a reminder, as it is sometimes easy to forget to take the preventer inhaler when asthma is well controlled and symptoms few and far between. Preventer inhalers are brown, orange, red or yellow.

There are three main types of preventer drugs:

- inhaled steroids
- sodium cromoglicate
- nedocromil.

Again, these come in a variety of different inhaler devices.

Inhaled steroids

The word 'steroid' conjures up disturbing pictures in many people's minds, and there is much misinformation circulating about these very effective drugs:

- These steroids are not the anabolic steroids used by body-builders and illegally by some athletes.

- The inhaled version, which is used as preventive treatment, is the same sort of drug as tablet steroids used for acute attacks of asthma and, for example, in some patients with arthritis.

- The dose of the inhaled drug is extremely small compared with that contained in steroid tablets. For instance, two puffs twice a day from an inhaler deliver anything from 20 to 400 micrograms of drug, depending on which is used. In acute asthma, six 5 milligram (mg) tablets of steroid will be given per day – 30,000 micrograms of drug, 75 to 1,500 times the inhaled dose.

- The side effects of inhaled steroids are few compared with those of oral steroids but, most importantly, are very much less than the dangers of undertreated asthma.

- Five per cent of patients on inhaled steroids will complain of a sore or dry mouth (sometimes this is caused by thrush), whilst a further five per cent may complain of some huskiness of voice; this is more important for some patients who use their voices a lot (such as teachers or telephone operators) than for others. The local effects of these inhalers can be minimised by mouth washing after each dose and by use of large-volume spacer devices, which act as 'reservoirs' and also markedly reduce the amount of drug deposited in the mouth.

- At higher doses (1,500 micrograms per day or more), particularly in older patients, side effects, such as easy bruising, may become apparent, along with an increase in the frequency of oral thrush and hoarseness. Cataracts may occur in some patients, but the suggestion that inhaled steroids cause osteoporosis (thinning of the bones) is debatable. Any such effects have to be balanced against the risks of undertreated asthma.

Inhalation of asthma drugs

Inhaling an asthma drug is the most effective treatment for the prevention and relief of asthma. The inhaler distributes the drug rapidly through the airways for instant relief of symptoms.

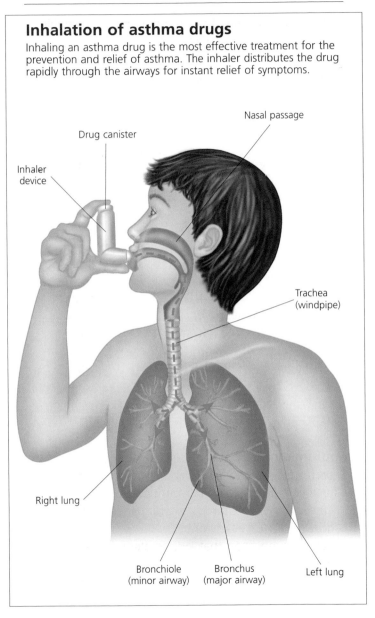

Drug canister

Nasal passage

Inhaler device

Trachea (windpipe)

Right lung

Bronchiole (minor airway)

Bronchus (major airway)

Left lung

- There is some evidence that in high doses a small proportion of children may show slight growth suppression with inhaled steroids but, interestingly, once the child with asthma reaches adult height, growth catch-up has virtually always occurred.

Chronic, undertreated asthma of childhood is more likely to cause growth suppression than inhaled steroids.

Inhaled steroids are very effective preventive drugs across the full spectrum of patients with asthma and are regarded as the preventive treatment of choice in most patients with asthma.

Combination inhalers (preventer and reliever)

There are now three inhalers – Seretide (combination of fluticasone and salmeterol), Symbicort (combination of budesonide and formoterol) and Fostair (combination of beclometasone and formoterol) – which contain both an inhaled steroid (preventer) and a long-acting inhaled bronchodilator (reliever). These reduce the hassle of taking two lots of inhalers and help in compliance with treatment. Generally, these combination inhalers are taken regularly, but Symbicort can be used on a variable-dose regimen according to symptoms.

Sodium cromoglicate

Sodium cromoglicate has been available for as long as inhaled steroids. It is a good form of prevention in the milder forms of childhood asthma, particularly in controlling exercise-induced symptoms. It needs to be used three or four times a day, a disadvantage when compared with inhaled steroids, but it can be used simply before exercise to prevent exercise-induced symptoms and has virtually no side effects.

Nedocromil (Tilade)

Nedocromil sodium has a preventive strength similar to that of low-dose inhaled steroids and comes as a mint-flavoured dry powder aerosol.

New drugs
Omalizumab (Xolair)

This revolutionary new drug is aimed at counteracting the effects of the allergy antibody immunoglobulin E (IgE). It comes as an injection given once every three weeks and is targeted at patients with severe allergic asthma. This shows great promise for patients with severe asthma, but will not be used in patients with milder disease. At present its use is limited in the UK because it is expensive.

Other preparations

There are two other groups of drugs used in the treatment of asthma:

- the theophyllines
- the leukotriene blockers.

Leukotriene blockers

The leukotriene blockers (Singulair, Accolate) are a relatively new form of asthma treatment. They are essentially preventive drugs but they do have slight bronchodilator effects. They appear to be of some benefit to a proportion of patients with a range of severities and in those with exercise-induced symptoms. There is some suggestion that symptoms of cough and sputum benefit more from these drugs. Although, in theory, these drugs may be of more benefit to patients with aspirin-sensitive asthma, not

The main types of inhaled asthma drugs

The majority of asthma drugs are inhaled. Relievers ease the symptoms of asthma once an attack has started.

Relievers	
Drug name	**Inhaler name**
Salbutamol	Ventolin Salbulin Salamol Airomir Evohaler
Terbutaline	Bricanyl
Salmeterol[a]	Serevent
Formoterol[a]	Foradil Oxis
Ipratropium	Atrovent
Tiotropium[b]	Spiriva
Salbutamol and ipratropium	Combivent[c]

[a] These are long-acting bronchodilators, the effect of which can last for as long as 12 hours.

[b] Tiotropium may last for 12 to 24 hours.

[c] Soon to be available only as a nebuliser solution.

The main types of inhaled asthma drugs (contd)

Preventers need to be used regularly to keep the symptoms of asthma under control.

Preventers	
Drug name	**Inhaler name**
Beclometasone	Asmabec Beclazone series AeroBec series Filair series Qvar series Clenil series
Budesonide	Pulmicort
Fluticasone[d]	Flixotide
Ciclesonide	Alvesco
Mometasone furoate	Asmanex
Sodium cromoglicate	Intal (puffer Spincaps) Cromolyn Nalcrom
Nedocromil	Tilade

[d] Dose for dose, fluticasone is twice as potent as beclometasone and budesonide.

everyone with this particular type of asthma appears to benefit; however, all should be given a trial of this particular form of drug. So far, these drugs seem to have relatively few side effects – reassuring for a tablet medication.

Theophyllines

The group of tablets known collectively as the theophyllines (for example, Uniphyllin Continus, Phyllocontin Continus, Nuelin SA) were originally used as bronchodilators, but tend to be used more in a preventive way now. They are probably used less than in the past because of the effectiveness and safety of inhaled steroids. They tend to cause nausea and headache in some patients, but have the advantage of being something that you just swallow – some people have difficulty mastering the use of an inhaler.

Emergency treatment

It is important when you have an acute attack that you seek urgent medical help. When an acute attack of asthma occurs, there are two mainstays of emergency treatment:

- big doses of reliever drug (often via a nebuliser)
- big doses of an anti-inflammatory drug (injected or oral steroids).

Some patients will be able to self-start emergency treatment with a nebuliser and/or a course of tablet steroids, but, for most patients who have not had a severe attack before, they should contact their GP as quickly as possible or attend the local accident and emergency department. Delay can be very dangerous and it is better to be safe than sorry.

Nebulisers

Nebulised drugs used in acute episodes are salbutamol (Ventolin), terbutaline (Bricanyl) and ipratropium (Atrovent). In some situations, ipratropium and salbutamol are given as a combined preparation (Combivent). Nebulisers should be obtained only after assessment by your doctor. The machine itself is a simple air compressor, which bubbles air through a solution of the drug, generating a mist that is inhaled through either a mask or a mouthpiece. The compressors themselves are not always available through the NHS in

How nebulisers work

The nebuliser is a simple air compressor. It bubbles air through a solution of the drug, generating a mist, which is inhaled through either a mask or a mouthpiece.

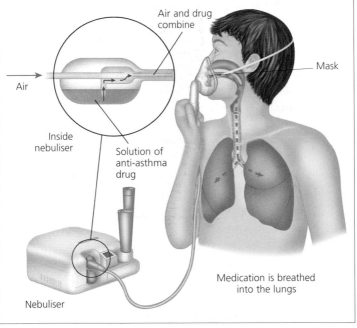

Air and drug combine

Mask

Air

Inside nebuliser

Solution of anti-asthma drug

Medication is breathed into the lungs

Nebuliser

every health district. You may have to buy your own or obtain one, often on a loan basis, through a charity such as Asthma UK (see page 107), with local branches that often run a nebuliser loan service.

There is, however, increasing evidence that larger doses of bronchodilators delivered by large-volume spacers (see below) are just as effective as nebulisers in acute asthma. This is particularly so in children because of the benefits of simplicity and cheapness.

Sometimes, nebulised drugs are prescribed to be used regularly in the patient with more severe asthma, but only when high doses of other treatments have proved inadequate. Nebulisers should not be used as an alternative to inhaled preventive treatment.

Delivery devices

In many patients, the simple metered dose inhalers (puffers) just cannot be used effectively. Poor inhaler technique can result in most of the drug escaping into the air through the top of the inhaler. The patient then believes that the inhaler is 'no good'.

If you are one of these patients, you can use another type of inhaler device that relies on your breath to suck the drug into the lung, as opposed to the puffer, where breathing in has to coincide with the squirt of the puffer.

The most frequently used type of 'breath-activated' device is the spacer, a large plastic 'balloon' which acts as a reservoir of drug from the puffer for the patient then to breathe in at the right moment. Spacers are made of brittle plastic and there is some evidence that they acquire quite a lot of static electrical charge, which makes the drug stick to the inside of the spacer, thus reducing the amount of drug getting into the lungs. The best plan is to wash the spacer once a week and allow it to drip dry. Rubbing with an antistatic cloth, such as can be found in Hi-Fi shops, can also help reduce this problem.

Other types of breath-activated devices are Rotahalers, Turbohalers, Diskhalers, Accuhalers, Clickhalers and Autohalers, all of which have different features, which suit some individuals more than others. In many cases it is clear that an individual patient is very much at home with a particular device.

Matching the patient with the right device is vital, as an acceptable device is more likely to be used at the right time and effectively. With the exception of the spacer devices, 'breath-activated devices' are more

Spacer devices

Allow the patient to concentrate on breathing in the medication rather than having to coordinate inhaling and pressing the inhaler button at the same time.

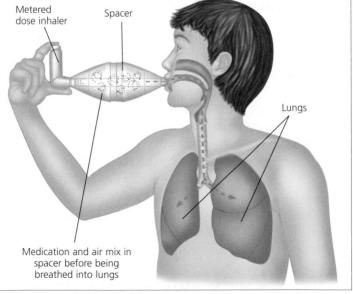

Metered dose inhaler

Spacer

Lungs

Medication and air mix in spacer before being breathed into lungs

The range of inhaler devices (not to scale)

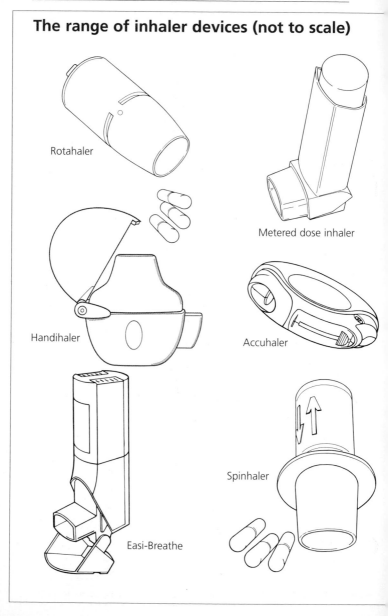

Rotahaler

Metered dose inhaler

Handihaler

Accuhaler

Easi-Breathe

Spinhaler

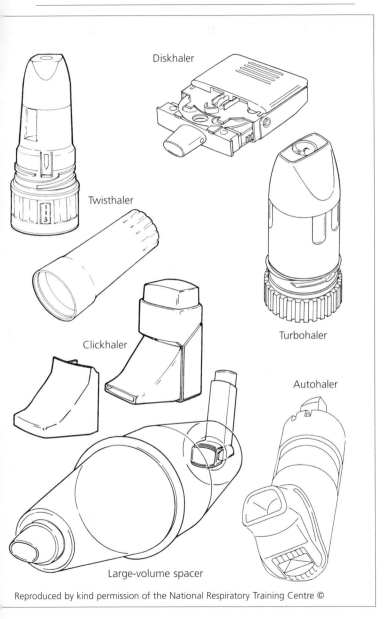

Diskhaler

Twisthaler

Turbohaler

Clickhaler

Autohaler

Large-volume spacer

expensive, although a correctly used 'expensive' device may, in the long term, be cheaper in terms of patient suffering than a poorly used 'cheap' device. Examples of these are seen on pages 58 and 59.

Phasing out of CFC-containing inhalers

Metered dose inhalers (puffers) contain CFCs which act as a propellant gas to help the jet of drug emerge. As a result of the effect of CFCs on the ozone layer, the Montreal Protocol states that those puffers that contain CFCs must be phased out as soon as possible. A number of companies are producing puffers that contain an alternative propellant, which does not have such an effect on the ozone layer. They look similar to existing puffers, but tend to have a more noticeable taste than the previous standard inhalers.

However, the drug in each inhaler is the same and they are just as effective in treating your asthma.

For reliever drugs, the non-CFC-containing inhalers are just as effective, but for one of the steroid inhalers (Qvar) the drug is twice as potent as the non-CFC preparation. Your pharmacist will be able to advise you about this.

KEY POINTS

- Drugs used in asthma treatment are relievers, preventers or emergency (reserve) drugs

- Inhaled steroids are the preventive treatment of choice in most patients with asthma

- The right combination of drug and inhaler device needs to be chosen for each patient

The management of asthma

Controlling asthma

The whole aim of managing asthma is to put you, the patient, in control of your asthma rather than have the asthma being in control of you. In patients who require only the occasional puff of their relief inhaler, this is straightforward, but, for patients with more significant asthma, management plans need to be developed and agreed by doctor and patient.

Although we have already said that asthma is a very personal condition and that what is right for one patient may not be right for another, nevertheless guidelines have been developed to help nurses and doctors in the management of all their patients with asthma. These were developed by a panel of experts representing the different groups involved in the management of asthma.

The guidelines are simple to use and are gradually being taken up by more doctors and respiratory nurse specialists. They are based on a series of upward steps in treatment to control asthma, and a series of downward steps when asthma appears to be in good control and when lower doses of treatment may be possible.

Before I describe the steps, just let me remind you about the importance of preventive measures, similar to those discussed in 'Prevention and self-help' (see page 35), which include control of allergens. It is very important to avoid certain drugs that cause asthma or make it worse (for example, aspirin – non-steroidal anti-inflammatory drugs or NSAIDs – or beta blockers, including beta-blocker eyedrops).

Even if you have been taking these medications for some time without problems, should you start to develop wheezy breathlessness, you should stop taking these tablets.

You should also stop drugs similar to aspirin, and seek alternatives (see 'Special forms of asthma', page 80). Discuss this with your doctor and pharmacist.

Guideline steps

The following guidelines are based on the British Asthma Guidelines, the latest version of which was published in 2008. These employ a graded method of controlling asthma symptoms using the minimum amount of drug.

Step 1

Most patients fit into this level. Patients are advised to use their relief inhaler as required. If your use of the relief inhaler is more than twice a week, or more than once a week for relief of night-time symptoms, you must see your doctor who will consider moving you to Step 2.

Step 2

If you are using a relief inhaler more than twice a week, or if for night-time symptoms more than once a week, you need a preventive inhaler, the choice of which is made by the doctor (see 'Drugs used in the treatment of asthma', page 46). This should result in you reducing the use of your inhaled reliever and improvement in your symptoms.

Step 3

If your symptoms persist, your doctor will also start you on a regular long-acting reliever, such as salmeterol, in addition to your other treatment. If your symptoms are not controlled with these inhalers, your doctor will consider increasing the dose of inhaled steroid and making other adjustments to your medication.

Steps to asthma control

These simple guidelines, developed by doctors and nurses involved in the treatment of asthma, allow for the minimum dose of the appropriate drug to be given so that the symptoms are adequately controlled.

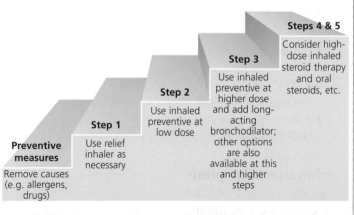

Steps 4 & 5
Consider high-dose inhaled steroid therapy and oral steroids, etc.

Step 3
Use inhaled preventive at higher dose and add long-acting bronchodilator; other options are also available at this and higher steps

Step 2
Use inhaled preventive at low dose

Step 1
Use relief inhaler as necessary

Preventive measures
Remove causes (e.g. allergens, drugs)

Subsequent steps (4 and 5)

If you are still having problems, the use of even higher doses of inhaled steroids, oral steroids and leukotriene receptor antagonists, among other treatment options, will be considered. At this stage, it is likely that you will be referred to a chest consultant for assessment, although some are referred at Step 3.

Step down

In medicine it is sometimes perhaps too easy to start a new treatment when symptoms do not come under control. It is not so easy to stop a treatment either because symptoms are well controlled or because the new drug had no extra benefit.

What to do during an asthma attack

- Remove yourself from any potential triggering environment such as the workplace or a smoky room
- Use reliever treatment according to your management plan
- Sit down, try to relax and stay calm. Think about something else
- If there is no response within 15 minutes repeat treatment
- If your management plan includes advice for starting oral steroids follow it
- If there is no response within a further 15 minutes, contact your GP, go to A&E or call an ambulance

Management plans

For many patients, a management plan can help greatly in controlling their asthma. This is a series of instructions

Sample asthma diary

Name:..

Record your answers to the following questions about your daily

	1 MON	2 TUES	3 WED	4 THUR	5 FRI
a. Did you cough today?					
b Did you wheeze today?					
c Were you short of breath today?					
d Did your asthma wake you in the night?					
e Were you off school or work today?					
f Has your asthma caused you to avoid any activities today?					

Record your peak-flow readings for each day of the week. You must take your readings every morning and evening. You should take three readings and record the best reading on the chart.

Time	am	pm	am	pm	am	pm	am	pm	am	pm
600										
550										
500										
450										
400										
350										
300										
250										
200										
150										
100										

Record how much (e.g. puffs or tablets) of each of your treatments you

Treatment name

1					
2					
3					

Sample asthma diary (contd)

Date:...

symptoms. If you have experienced the symptom tick the box.

6 SAT		7 SUN		8 MON		9 TUE		10 WED		11 THUR		12 FRI		13 SAT		14 SUN	

am	pm	am	pm	am	pm	am	pm	am	pm	am	pm	am	pm	am	pm	am	pm

have taken during the day (24 hours).

on what to do when your asthma starts to slip or in situations in which your asthma may be thought likely to worsen. There are two types of management plan.

Peak-flow-based management plans

The peak-flow meter is simple to use and to read. A short sharp blow will record the maximum rate at which air can be blown out of your lungs. Usually, three attempts are made, and you record the highest. Recording a value twice a day (on waking and on going to bed) is usually sufficient, although sometimes your doctor will ask for more frequent recordings.

With a management plan based on peak flow, you will be provided with a peak-flow meter and a chart on which to record the peak-flow readings. You may also be provided with two target values. These will vary, often considerably, between patients, and will be personalised by the GP or respiratory nurse to suit your particular pattern of peak-flow readings.

The first level is the target peak flow, which is usually 70 to 80 per cent of best. If your peak flow is above this value, you need not adjust your treatment, but, if your peak flow falls below this over a 24-hour period, you should double your inhaled preventive treatment until your peak flows have climbed above the target peak flow, and remained there for two or three days. This system works for many, but not all, individuals, and your doctor may decide that this approach is unsuitable for you.

The second value is usually about 50 to 60 per cent of best. At this level you should use a course of oral steroids. You may be allowed to take this course of action yourself, although some doctors prefer to see the patient if oral steroids are needed.

A final threshold is set, at which you should seek medical assistance as soon as possible, from either your GP or the local accident and emergency department. This level of peak flow will be set by the doctor.

The chart for recording peak flows may be either a series of columns on which the recordings are written, usually twice a day, or a graph-like chart to plot the values. Some patients prefer this second form of chart because the variation in levels of peak flow can be more easily appreciated.

Case history 1: peak-flow-based plan

William had always been a difficult little lad, and not just as far as his asthma was concerned. He tended to take his inhalers only when he felt the need and consequently was constantly missing school. By the time he had reached secondary school, with no sign of his asthma abating, his GP decided to try to establish a management plan.

For the first time, William started to record his peak-flow readings at home on waking and on going to bed. The peak-flow meter stayed by his bed and his parents were able to check that he was recording the values on his chart. Somewhat to his surprise, William found that his peak-flow readings varied considerably, dropping as low as 150 on waking but reaching 270 by evening time.

The penny having dropped, he began to take his inhaled preventive more regularly and the peak-flow variation became less marked, the readings also increasing somewhat to settle between 300 and 350. By that stage he was taking two puffs night and morning of inhaled steroid and had begun to use the relief inhaler much less frequently.

The GP then gave him a target peak flow of 275, advising him to double his preventer if the values dropped below this over a 24-hour period, and keeping at the higher dose until he was above target for at least three days.

A second threshold was given of 175, below which William knew to contact his GP for a course of oral steroids. In the event, oral steroids did not become necessary. William began to notice the benefits of his regular preventive therapy and over the subsequent year had to increase his inhaled steroids (peak flows fell below 275) on only three occasions.

Managing your child's asthma

- Ensure that you recognise what triggers your child's asthma and avoid where possible
- Ban smoking anywhere in the house! This will have the benefit of improved health in those who stop in addition to the benefit to the child
- Ensure that you understand your child's medication and how and when it should be used
- Ensure that your child does take his or her treatment!
- If your child is old enough ensure that he or she is aware how to use the medication
- It is worthwhile discussing your child's asthma with your child's school to ensure that they are aware of the issues surrounding your child's asthma in particular
- Discuss the use of a management plan with your GP or hospital doctor or asthma nurse and follow it if provided with one

Symptom-based management plans

The same concept as that of a peak-flow-based plan operates here, except that certain levels of symptoms are used as prompts for changes in treatment as opposed to changes in peak-flow values.

Case history 2: symptom-based plan

Jacky had not got on well with peak-flow measurements. They did not seem to tell her much more about her asthma than her symptoms did and they began to be a pain to do, being 'just for the sake of the doctor', as she saw it. Luckily, the GP became aware of this and suggested a switch to a symptom-based plan. By doubling her inhaled preventive if she used more than three puffs of relief inhaler a day over two successive days, or when she started a cold, or if she started to wake at night with symptoms, her asthma was more effectively controlled. If doubling the inhaled preventive didn't stop her symptoms, she knew that she had to go to her GP for reassessment, although if she had to do that she did measure her peak flow a few times before the consultation 'just to see'. This helped the GP believe that she was managing her asthma sensibly.

Exhaled nitric oxide

Recently, it has been shown that the amount of the gas nitric oxide (NO) in exhaled breath seems to be a marker of whether or not someone's asthma is well controlled. It is relatively early days yet, but there is some hope to think that this might prove useful in assessing asthma control. At present, this is likely to be a test done only in the clinic or GP surgery, and is largely a research tool.

Choosing a plan

Some patients seem better suited to peak-flow-based plans, others to symptom-based plans, and the decision which to use is often based on a number of factors. Some individuals are either unable or unwilling to use either type but, where asthma appears to remain poorly controlled, every effort will be made by the doctor or nurse to find a system that will help the patient manage the asthma better. Sometimes a combination of symptoms and peak flow can be used for certain individuals. Both plans will include advice to anticipate problems such as colds or exposure to known allergens. If you develop the early symptoms of a cold, your doctor may advise you to double the dose of your inhaled preventive treatment and continue for at least a week until the symptoms pass, when you can resume the original dose. Some patients need inhaled steroids only for colds and they should be advised to start at the slightest beginnings of a cold and continue for two weeks, unless their asthma still continues to cause problems, in which case they should stay on their preventive treatment and contact their GP.

Clinic nurses

Asthma clinics have been set up in many GP surgeries, run either by the GP or by the practice nurse. Many are run by nurses who have been specifically trained in the management of asthma at recognised training centres. Their role in the management of asthma is very important and they have helped to provide a much better service for the patient with asthma in general practice, with fewer referrals to hospital from practices where such a system operates and more appropriate referrals when the patient is running into problems.

Asthma nurse

Many doctors' practices now have a fully trained asthma nurse to advise asthma patients and manage the treatment of their condition.

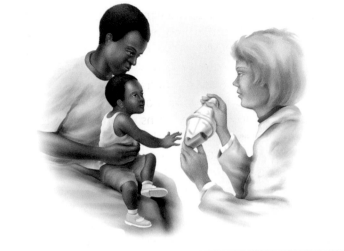

Often, the asthma nurse will see patients with asthma more than the doctor will, releasing the doctor for other patients, but the nurse knows very well when the doctor needs to see the patient if things are not going well. It ought to be the aim of all general practices to set up an asthma clinic run by a fully trained asthma nurse.

KEY POINTS

■ Guidelines have been developed to help nurses and doctors provide optimal management of all patients with asthma using a series of treatment steps

■ One way of giving patients good control over their asthma is to provide them with management plans

■ Management plans may either be peak-flow based or symptom based

■ Many GP surgeries have set up asthma clinics, often run by specially trained asthma nurses

Asthma in elderly people

Who gets asthma?

Asthma tends to be regarded as a condition of the young, particularly children, and indeed it is very much more common in children, as we have seen. As these patients become older, some have persistent symptoms, some have only minor symptoms and some have lost their symptoms to all intents and purposes.

There are some patients who develop asthma for the first time in their later years. It is often believed that these patients are more likely to have more severe asthma and to have to take oral steroids. It is also believed that allergies are less likely to be found as the cause. Although these beliefs are true up to a point, it is important to realise that there is always a great overlap in patterns of asthma throughout the ages. Yet, again, it bears repeating that each patient needs to be assessed as an individual.

Symptoms

The symptoms in the older patient are identical to those in the younger patient with asthma except that breathlessness, especially on exertion, is quite common. This is often due to the fact that many people over the age of 60 have, at some stage, smoked cigarettes and are left with an amount of irreversible bronchial tube narrowing. This means that exertion will cause breathlessness more quickly in some individuals.

Problems can occur when an older patient complains of chest tightness on exertion. As heart disease is common in this age group and angina can cause this very same symptom, delay in diagnosis – both of angina and of asthma – can occur.

Case history: late-onset asthma

Tom, an 82-year-old man, went to his GP with a six-month history of episodes of breathlessness. Sometimes these came on out of the blue and sometimes when he exerted himself. He did not feel that he was wheezy but did admit that he got a tight feeling in his chest, particularly when he got breathless on exertion.

Quite rightly, the GP's first impression in a man of this age was that this was likely to be the result of heart disease, but treatment for angina had no effect. He was sent to a consultant at hospital who felt that late-onset asthma needed to be ruled out, although he was fairly certain that this was an unlikely diagnosis. To the consultant's surprise and delight, the peak-flow readings recorded assiduously by the patient showed the typical variation seen in asthma, and prescription of anti-asthma medication resulted in great improvements in his symptoms.

The patient's reaction on realising that he had asthma was interesting in that his major reaction was one of anger.

'Why me? I've never smoked and always looked after myself. There's no one in the family who has suffered from asthma. Why me?'

Explanation and reassurance and the fact that, on two puffs twice a day of inhaled steroid, he improved greatly did relieve his anger. He is now able to garden as he did before with only the occasional need to use his relief inhaler.

What is the treatment?

Again, treatment of asthma in the older patient with asthma is the same, and follows the same steps, as in the younger patient. Where problems can occur is in the manageability of the inhaler devices. The Rotacap dry powder system can be very fiddly for an arthritic hand and even the metered dose inhaler (puffer) can be impossible to use for patients with stiff or painful hands. Attachments are available to make the puffer usable by these patients (for example, Haleraid, made by Allen & Hanburys and available on request from chemists), but often the simple expedient of a large-volume spacer will ease the problem, although other handier breath-activated devices (see pages 56–60) should be considered. It is really a matter of tailoring the inhaler device to the patient.

As age creeps up, patients often find themselves on a variety of different pills, potions and other medications for a range of conditions. This can often be very confusing and it is the doctor's responsibility to keep the 'regimen' of treatment as simple as possible. It may even be necessary to sacrifice the ideal treatment just to ensure that the most important treatments are taken.

Side effects of medication for older patients

Side effects of any form of treatment are more common in the older patient. In the person with more severe asthma, the side effects of oral steroids can be severe, particularly osteoporosis and skin changes, with easy bruising, skin thinning and poor wound healing. Patients taking high-dose inhaled steroids (more than 1,500 micrograms per day) can also develop these skin changes, although to a less dramatic degree.

What is the outlook?

Asthma starting in later years is unlikely to leave the patient, who usually has found an unwanted companion for life. The severity does not necessarily get worse, however, and good treatment properly applied will be very effective in controlling symptoms.

Each individual will have his or her own targets or needs. For some it will simply be the ability to potter in the garden, which their untreated asthma may have stopped them doing. Others may wish to be able to go rambling again, or to be able to do their own shopping or go to the pub for a drink with their friends. Success is achieving their own target, not necessarily increasing the dose of inhaler up and up to try to achieve an improvement that the patient may not want or need, or realistically be able to achieve.

As I mentioned earlier, deaths from asthma increased in elderly people through the 1990s, although the reasons for this are not clear. I suspect that many would have been regarded as having died of bronchitis in days gone by (and, indeed, some of these deaths from asthma more recently may be due more to chronic bronchitis). So we must not be complacent in our attempts to prevent death from asthma at whatever age it may be causing problems.

The outlook for the older patient with asthma should be regarded positively. The treatment is safe and effective, although the more severely affected patient may need to find a balance between symptoms of asthma and side effects of drugs.

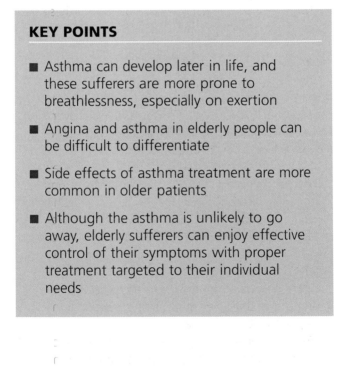

KEY POINTS

■ Asthma can develop later in life, and these sufferers are more prone to breathlessness, especially on exertion

■ Angina and asthma in elderly people can be difficult to differentiate

■ Side effects of asthma treatment are more common in older patients

■ Although the asthma is unlikely to go away, elderly sufferers can enjoy effective control of their symptoms with proper treatment targeted to their individual needs

Special forms of asthma

In many cases, the cause of asthma is unknown. In others, however, an allergen will commonly trigger an attack. Other special forms of asthma include nocturnal asthma, aspirin-sensitive asthma and brittle asthma.

Allergic asthma

If an allergy or more than one allergy has been identified as being potentially important on the basis of your history, it is sometimes necessary to do further tests to confirm this and to identify the allergen. The test is simple and takes about half an hour to complete.

A series of drops of various solutions of substances, which are known to cause allergic reactions (for example, house dust mite, grass pollen, tree pollen, cat dander, etc.), are placed on the forearm. Using small needle points, the skin surface is then gently pierced through each droplet to allow the substance to get under the skin. After 15 minutes or so, local reactions can occur, which look like small areas of nettle rash

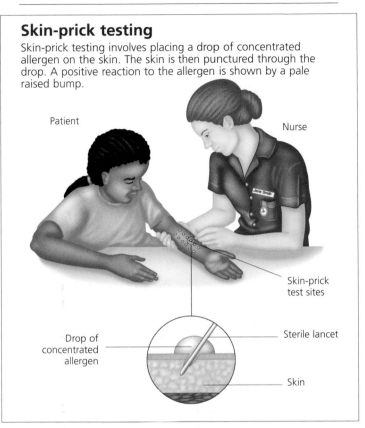

Skin-prick testing

Skin-prick testing involves placing a drop of concentrated allergen on the skin. The skin is then punctured through the drop. A positive reaction to the allergen is shown by a pale raised bump.

Patient

Nurse

Skin-prick test sites

Drop of concentrated allergen

Sterile lancet

Skin

and usually itch. The needle pricks themselves are not painful – just a tiny scratch – but the itching can be maddening and lasts half an hour or so.

The size of the reaction (or weal) can be measured for each allergen, which gives an idea, not only of what you are allergic to, but also of how allergic you may be to each allergen. Sometimes this is helpful in management because it could tell you which triggers to avoid and could identify things that may turn out to be not so important.

The danger is that small reactions may not be important but sometimes, as a result, patients will then take unnecessary actions. I have seen the occasional patient on extraordinary and unnecessary diets, based on weakly positive skin tests, which have not helped their asthma. This is not always the case: everyone is an individual and his or her needs must be individually addressed.

Desensitisation

If you are shown to be allergic to a particular allergen (for example, cat or rabbit), you can't avoid contact with these animals and your asthma continues to be poorly controlled by the usual treatment regimens, desensitisation may be considered. This should be done only at specialist centres and should be undertaken only for one allergen at a time. Certainly, for patients with asthma, they should be conducted only at a hospital because there have been many examples of severe reactions to desensitisation, with attacks of asthma needing hospital admission and even causing deaths. For hay fever alone the dangers are less, but for asthma great care needs to be taken.

The process involves a series of injections of small amounts of the substance to which you are allergic, usually under the skin of the upper arm. Very, very small quantities are used to start with, the concentrations increasing week by week or day by day ('rush' immunotherapy) to avoid severe allergic reactions. There are different timescales over which the courses of injections are undertaken before a course is considered complete, and this will be up to the centre involved and your needs. Small local reactions (a reddening of the skin at the injection site) are not infrequent, but these settle quickly on the day of the injection. Once the course is complete, boosters can be given at varying intervals if the course has been thought to be successful.

In the UK, desensitisation for asthma is only rarely undertaken, largely because of the fear of bad reactions, but also because many doctors do not believe that this treatment works. If you wish to talk further about whether this might be of use (and it is likely to be useful in only a minority of patients with asthma), then ask your GP for a referral to a centre with experience in this area. A list of specialist centres can be obtained from Allergy UK (see 'Useful addresses' on page 106).

Nocturnal asthma

Night-time asthma is often regarded as a particular type of asthma. In fact, waking at night with asthma is an indication of asthma that is poorly controlled overall and applies to any patient with any type of asthma. In most cases, appropriate treatment will overcome the problem but some patients are more difficult to control. In these patients, factors such as acid reflux (stomach acid coming back into the chest at night and causing irritation) may be a cause and need treatment. Some drugs, such as theophyllines and the long-acting inhaled bronchodilators, are often helpful in controlling symptoms of nocturnal asthma.

Aspirin-sensitive asthma

Aspirin sensitivity occurs in around five per cent of adult patients with asthma. It is very rare in children. These patients are nearly always negative on skin testing for allergens and may suffer from nasal polyps on a recurring basis. If you are such a patient, you

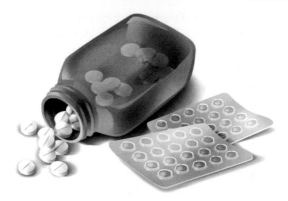

Patients with aspirin-sensitive asthma can die from unwittingly swallowing a preparation containing aspirin.

must avoid all aspirin-containing drugs, including a wide range of arthritis drugs such as ibuprofen, diclofenac and indometacin (collectively the non-steroidal anti-inflammatory drugs or NSAIDs). If you are unsure whether a particular drug might interfere with your asthma, ask your GP or your pharmacist. Patients with aspirin-sensitive asthma can die from unwittingly swallowing a preparation containing aspirin. Although the treatment usually simply involves avoidance, desensitisation can be done with success, but this is available only in specialist centres.

Desensitisation for this form of asthma is done using small doses of aspirin given orally, the patient being closely monitored at hospital with repeated breathing tests for some hours after each dose. It is time-consuming in the first instance, but is worthwhile for some.

Brittle asthma

Brittle asthma is a rare form of asthma. The patient

suffers from sudden severe attacks, sometimes in spite of apparently being very well controlled. Others develop attacks on a background of asthma, which doctor and patient have great difficulty in controlling on a day-to-day basis. These patients keep being admitted to hospital and are at increased risk of dying from their asthma. Allergy seems to be more common in these patients and sometimes their acute attacks follow inhaling or eating something to which they are allergic. Their asthma often puts a huge strain on both the patient and family, and psychological factors seem to be very important – but whether the asthma causes the psychological disturbance or the other way around is a moot point.

Treatment is extremely difficult and patients should be managed by chest specialists with an interest in the more severe forms of asthma.

KEY POINTS

■ A history of allergy may lead to the need for confirmatory tests to identify the allergen

■ Desensitisation in asthma patients can be dangerous and should be done only in hospital

■ Night-time asthma suggests that asthma is poorly controlled

■ Individuals with asthma who are sensitive to aspirin should avoid all aspirin-containing drugs. Ask your GP or pharmacist if you are in doubt

■ Patients with brittle asthma should be managed by chest specialists with an interest in the more severe forms of asthma

Occupational asthma

Workplace exposure

Asthma that develops as a result of exposure to a substance or substances at work is regarded as occupational asthma. The exposure may act as an inducer of asthma, where the substance sensitises the patient to such an extent that further reactions are caused at every subsequent exposure.

Alternatively, the substance may act as an inciter, inducing attacks in patients who already have asthma, which did not necessarily arise originally as a result of the exposure.

Causes

There are over 400 known causes of occupational asthma, many of them obscure, but some of them occurring in very familiar types of work. They include isocyanates (the hardener in paints used by car body paint sprayers), epoxy resins and flour (baker's asthma).

A list of the more common causes of occupational asthma is shown opposite, along with the jobs with which these forms are usually associated.

Common causes of occupational asthma

Some of the most common causes of occupational asthma are shown in this chart, together with the jobs in which you are most likely to encounter each substance.

Causes/substances	Occupations
Isocyanates	Paint, varnish and some plastics workers
Flour	Bakery/catering trades
Colophony	Solderers
Animal urine	Laboratory workers, animal breeders
Epoxy resins	Occupations involved with adhesives/varnishes
Chromium	Tanning, electroplating
Enzymes	Detergent production, drug/food technology
Hardwood dusts	Millers, joiners, carpenters
Nickel	Electroplating
Dyes	Dye manufacture
Antibiotics	Drug manufacturing
Grain mites	Farmers

Frequency

It has been estimated that between 10 and 15 per cent of all new cases occurring in adult life are due to that individual's occupation, but this figure may be an underestimate of the true incidence. As patients, employers and doctors are often unaware of the possibility that occupational factors could be important, many cases go undiagnosed, which, in some individuals, may be a problem because continued exposure to certain substances can lead to irreversible changes in the airways.

Diagnosis

The first clue comes from the patient's history. If your symptoms get better at the weekend or when you are away from work for longer periods, such as holidays, this suggests that something at work may be affecting your asthma. Not all who give such a history do have occupational asthma and, equally, some who don't give such a history do end up with a diagnosis of occupational asthma. However, such a history should result in referral to a chest specialist for further investigations.

After you have been referred to the hospital or chest clinic, the specialist will ask you to record your peak flows regularly, maybe as frequently as every two hours, both when at work and when away from work, to look for recognisable patterns of change in the peak-flow readings that would support the diagnosis.

Case history: spray-paint allergy

Brian is 32 years old and has worked in the car industry for 10 years since he had a spell in the Army, where he had begun to learn his trade. For the first four years, he had done various jobs around the factory, but he was switched to the paint shop at the age of 26. Although he used to smoke 10 to 15 cigarettes a day, his only problem up to that time had been the occasional bout of winter bronchitis.

During the winter before last, he had what he thought to be another attack of bronchitis with cough and wheeze, but on this occasion the symptoms persisted and began to wake him at night. He went to his GP who prescribed him another course of antibiotics and told him he really must stop smoking. This had no effect and his wheezing now began to be obvious on even modest exertion. The GP felt he might have asthma and treated him to some effect shortly before Brian went off on holiday the following Easter.

While away, Brian began to feel very much better and even stopped using his inhalers, but as soon as he went back to work his asthma returned with a vengeance. Suspecting that his improvement away from work might imply an occupational aspect to his asthma, his GP referred him to the local chest clinic where serial peak-flow readings showed the typical pattern of work-related asthma. Luckily, the firm for which Brian worked was a large concern and they provided him with a very effective protective hood. Since then his asthma has been much easier to control, and he has been able to continue work in a job in which he has become skilled and well paid.

Confirming the diagnosis

Occasionally, where there still may be doubt about an occupational origin for your asthma, you may be 'challenged' in the laboratory to the suspected substance under carefully supervised conditions. If you worsen when exposed to the suspect agent but not when exposed – on another day – to another substance not thought to be involved, this will usually clinch the diagnosis. This is a time-consuming process, as you may have to have a week off work, with repeated series of breathing tests being performed after different exposures in a specially constructed laboratory. There are relatively few of these centres in the UK.

The patient's future

Some people with occupational asthma are forced to leave their job, often because their asthma is too difficult to control while they continue to be exposed. In many cases, the factory management are either unable or unwilling to improve factory conditions. Some patients are repositioned within the company in a different job where exposure to the offending substance does not occur. Many, however, continue to work and to be exposed, which may be acceptable in some cases if their asthma can be controlled by medication. For those who are forced to leave their employment or are sacked because of poor work attendance, compensation is available for most people through the Industrial Injuries Disablement system.

Ask at your Benefits Office or Job Centre for form BI 100 (OA) and a reply envelope, and fill in the form. More information can be found in leaflet DB 1, which can be obtained from the same place. If you have any further queries, the staff at the Benefits Agency will be able to help you.

Sometimes, claims for compensation have to go through the courts, which invariably takes time, but may be the only way a skilled worker who has lost a well-paid job can be adequately compensated.

KEY POINTS

■ Asthma symptoms that improve at the weekend or during holidays suggest an occupational cause

■ The clue usually comes from the history, but the diagnosis may need to be confirmed in the laboratory

■ Compensation for those who have to leave their employment is available for most people through the Industrial Injuries Disablement system

Complementary treatments

Clinical trials

There is considerable interest in the role of alternative or complementary therapies for the treatment of asthma. This is due to worries about the side effects of conventional medical treatment and a belief that 'natural substances' are better for asthma than drugs.

Although virtually all the available standard treatments for asthma have been proven in properly controlled trials of efficacy, only rarely have complementary approaches been so assessed, although some complementary therapies have now been through trials for a range of conditions, with variable results. This is why many doctors pour scorn on such forms of treatment. Yet complementary practitioners often quote anecdotal stories of benefit and maintain that consistent successes over many years show that their treatment works. This has resulted in a polarisation of belief between those who feel that conventional medicine is the only suitable treatment

Complementary therapies

Acupuncture

There is no doubt that acupuncture has found more acceptance in medical circles than have other forms of complementary therapy, particularly with regard to pain relief. It is also one of the few alternative approaches that has been properly tested in clinical tests in asthma. Minor benefits have been shown in mild asthma, but acupuncture has not been shown to be of help in patients with more severe asthma.

The Buteyko technique

This technique has been suggested as a treatment for asthma, but it more likely treats the 'hyperventilation' (excessively fast breathing) seen in some individuals with asthma. This technique may reduce symptoms in some but does not affect the underlying asthma.

Homoeopathy

There are homoeopathic remedies for chronic asthma that are claimed to work. However, the more strict homoeopaths tell me that their treatment will be effective only if the patient stops taking his or her conventional medication – something that I could never condone.

Hypnosis

Some patients claim great benefits from hypnosis, particularly in the way that they are able to cope

Complementary therapies (contd)

with acute attacks or worsening asthma. For those who believe in this approach, it may be of help, but, as with homoeopathy, it would be very helpful to see properly conducted trials of its effect, which, to date, are lacking.

Herbalism

Herbalists often target their therapy on symptoms rather than the condition itself. So, if cough is a predominant symptom of asthma, specific attempts to reduce sputum production will be made, often with suggestions for dietary control.

Speleotherapy

I have put this in more to make a point than to recommend it as a possible approach for the British patient with asthma.

Speleotherapy involves patients spending time, often quite long periods, underground in caves! It appears to work, almost certainly because the patient has been removed from exposure to the house dust mite and other allergens. It is similar to the finding that spending time at altitude helps the person with bad asthma – again as a result of reduced exposure to the house dust mite.

So environmental control, when it involves removing the patient from exposure to allergens, can help. The problem is finding such an environment to live in!

and those who regard conventional treatment as verging on the poisonous! I believe that the truth lies between these two extremes although, predictably, I place more belief in standard medical treatment for asthma.

Looking at the 'whole' person

Nevertheless, the patient needs to be regarded as a whole and not just as 'a case of asthma': his or her beliefs need to be considered and discussed and, very often, where beliefs are strongly held on both sides, compromises can be made or deals can be struck. It must always be remembered that the aim is to control asthma or at least reduce it to an acceptable level in the patient's eyes.

Conventional therapy must remain the mainstay for the treatment of asthma in the long term but, in some patients who wish to explore alternative therapies, the benefits may be significant.

One important point that must be made is that patients should not simply stop their conventional treatment and switch to an alternative therapy. This has resulted in marked deterioration in some patients who have tried such a wholesale change.

Whether any benefit from complementary measures is the result of an effect of belief on such a suggestible condition as asthma or of a direct effect on asthmatic airways is open to debate; perhaps that debate should be encouraged at a more scientific level than it has been in the past.

KEY POINTS

■ Some complementary therapies do appear to help some patients. Whether this is the result of their belief in the effectiveness of the alternative approach or of a direct effect on asthmatic airways has not been established

■ With the exception of acupuncture, the benefits of complementary approaches have rarely been tested in properly controlled trials

The future

So what does the future hold for the person with asthma? First, there is no doubt that asthma is not going to disappear. It is very common and is likely to remain at current levels for the foreseeable future. Deaths from asthma will still occur.

This all sounds very pessimistic, but there are a number of lights in the darkness which potentially hold out hope for patients with asthma.

Prevention
It is likely that we will become better at controlling exposure to allergens, and this will be especially important in the first five years of life, when sensitisation to the house dust mite in particular occurs. Such control will require considerable effort on the part of the individual patient or parent! What doctors have to do is come up with a package of control measures that are practical and not cripplingly expensive. So far, they have fallen short of this ideal.

Other environmental control measures are needed, notably a reduction in parental smoking, which is so important in the development of asthma in children. There is no easy way to achieve this. Reduction in relevant occupational exposures is being practised more and more, while improvements in outdoor air quality should reduce asthma attacks.

Treatment

Producing a new drug for any condition is a long and costly business, requiring stringent animal and human studies that have to satisfy the Commission on Human Medicines and the National Institute for Health and Clinical Excellence (NICE) that the drug is both useful and safe. Only then will they provide a product licence for the drug.

So what new drugs are getting through this series of hoops that might be of help to patients with asthma in the near future?

New drugs

Interestingly, some of the new drugs on the horizon are in tablet form, as is the case with the leukotriene blockers (see page 51). After all, inhalers can be a nuisance – they are often tricky to use well and only rarely get used as regularly as doctors would like to believe.

These new drugs, whether inhaled, oral or injected, are being studied at present and we have yet to determine whether they will benefit people with all forms of asthma or only certain groups. Certainly, they have the potential to make asthma control easier, more acceptable and with few side effects.

It is likely that, in the longer term, very specific treatments, perhaps aimed at particular groups of people with asthma, will become available. Whether these will be in inhaled or tablet form will depend on

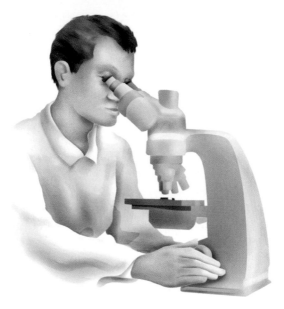

Successfully developing and releasing a new drug on to the market is an extremely expensive and time-consuming process.

many things, not the least of which will be what patients prefer!

Other drugs aimed, among other things, at specific chemicals that cause asthmatic inflammation are being tested (for example, anti-interleukin drugs) with, again, promising early results.

Gene therapy

Although great strides are being made in unravelling the genetics of asthma, particularly with respect to allergy, the possibility of gene therapy is a long way off.

Potentially, this could have almost the greatest effect on asthma but there are many hurdles, both ethical and scientific, to be overcome before that time.

Conclusion

I am optimistic about the future for the person with asthma. The development of drugs with fewer side effects or, better still, improved ways of preventing asthma or asthma attacks will come, and will reduce the discomfort that you and other asthma sufferers endure today.

KEY POINTS

- New drugs are being tested that have the potential to make asthma control easier, more acceptable and with fewer side effects

- Asthma will not be 'eradicated'; however, attempts to prevent rather than treat asthma should be effective in asthma control in the UK

Questions and answers

Will the asthma go?

This is the question most commonly asked by parents about their child with asthma. Most children of primary school age appear to lose their asthma, often in their teens, so a condition that is more common in boys becomes slightly more common in women. This is not to say that the asthma has disappeared for ever, as a proportion of patients suffer a relapse in later life – in women this is often around the time of the menopause. Sometimes, the symptoms of the newly returned asthma are different from those experienced as a child – wheezing will often be more common in childhood, and breathlessness and chest tightness more common in adulthood.

Most people who develop asthma in adult life will retain it to a greater or lesser degree for the rest of their lives. It is not clear what proportion who develop asthma in adulthood lose it, but a reasonable estimate would be around only 20 per cent.

Will the asthma or treatment damage the lungs?
Patients believe that 'the lungs' are different from 'the tubes' whereas the tubes are a part of the lungs.

The worry about long-term damage is, however, a real one. Undertreated, asthma can lead to irreversible narrowing of the airways because the inflammation is not being controlled. Similarly, patients who smoke and don't use their preventive inhaler regularly may develop quite severe irreversible damage to their lungs.

The treatment for asthma does not damage the lungs, although steroid tablets can cause many other side effects, as discussed on pages 46–54.

Taken overall, the risks of damage to the individual are greater with untreated asthma than when the asthma is controlled.

Will the treatment wear off?
The drug treatment for asthma does not wear off. If you find that your relief inhaler is becoming less effective, this is far more likely to be due to worsening asthma than the drug itself having no effect. Perhaps the prescribed dose is too small or, because the airways are narrower as the asthma worsens, less will be getting to the lower airways. If you find that your treatment is becoming less effective, it is essential that you go to your doctor for reassessment. It is not true that taking a certain dose of an inhaler will lead to you needing a progressively higher dose as the years go by.

Is asthma catching?
No it is not. Asthma is not an infectious disease and cannot be caught from another person.

Are nebulisers dangerous?

A nebuliser is a powerful way of delivering drugs to the lungs and is therefore used only in the patient with more severe asthma. Nevertheless, there are some patients using nebuliser therapy for whom other forms of treatment haven't been fully explored. When used only for acute attacks, nebulisers can save lives and admission to hospital.

The danger comes when too much reliance is placed on the 'all-powerful' nebuliser and, instead of seeking medical help, the patient self-administers repeated nebulised doses. This can lead to a very severe, even life-threatening, episode, which could have been avoided had the patient gone to the accident and emergency department or contacted his or her GP.

Once a patient is established on regular nebulised therapy, clearly his or her asthma is bad. Many will never be able to stop the treatment, unless a new treatment, which may be perfect for them, comes along. Occasionally, changes in circumstances, such as a move to a different part of the country, or removal from an occupational cause, can result in marked improvement in their asthma and they may then not need to use their nebuliser.

Again, as with other forms of inhaled therapy, using nebulised therapy under good supervision will not mean that you will need higher and higher doses as the years go by. If that appears to be happening it is more likely to be a result of the asthma itself worsening than an effect of the nebulised drug.

I am thinking of becoming pregnant. How and what should I do with my preventer/reliever medications?

The risk of an asthma attack is far greater than any

potential risk from medications. All inhaled therapy is entirely safe to both mother and child during pregnancy. There is a small risk that courses of oral steroids taken during the first three months of pregnancy increase the chances of having a baby with a harelip or a cleft palate – all the more reason for maintaining inhaled therapy to prevent the need for oral steroids.

The same principles apply to breast-feeding although again oral steroids will be transmitted in breast milk, as will the oral theophylline group of drugs. It would be probably sensible to avoid using oral theophyllines (Nuelin, Uniphylline, see page 54) to avoid the small risk of the baby having side effects such as nausea.

Useful addresses

We have included the following organisations because, on preliminary investigation, they may be of use to the reader. However, we do not have first-hand experience of each organisation and so cannot guarantee the organisation's integrity. The reader must therefore exercise his or her own discretion and judgement when making further enquiries.

Allergy UK (British Allergy Foundation)

3 White Oak Square, London Road
Swanley, Kent BR8 7AG
Helpline: 01322 619898
Website:www.allergyuk.org

Encompasses all types of allergies and offers information, quarterly newsletter and support network; translation cards for travel abroad.

Anaphylaxis Campaign

PO Box 275, Farnborough

Hants GU14 6SX
Tel: 01252 546100
Helpline: 01252 542029
Website: www.anaphylaxis.org.uk

Campaigns for better awareness of life-threatening
allergic reactions from food and drug allergies to bee
and wasp stings. Produces a wide range of educational
news sheets and videos and has extensive support
network. Send an SAE for information.

Asthma UK

England, Wales and N. Ireland
Summit House, 70 Wilson Street
London EC2A 2DB
Tel: 020 7786 4900
Helpline: 0845 701 0203 (Mon–Fri, 9am–5pm)
Website: www.asthma.org.uk

Provides a wide range of information for people with
asthma and their families. Helpline staffed by specialist
asthma nurses. Has some support groups and funds
medical research. Offers supervised holidays for young
people with asthma.The following are branches of
Asthma UK, providing a wide range of information for
people with asthma and their families. Funds medical
research.

Asthma UK Cymru

3rd floor, Eastgate House
34–43 Newport Road
Cardiff CF24 0AB
Tel: 02920 435 400

Asthma UK Northern Ireland
The Mount, 2 Woodstock Link
Belfast BT6 8DD
Tel: 02890 737290

Asthma UK Scotland
4 Queen Street
Edinburgh EH2 1JE
Tel: 0131 226 2544

Benefits Enquiry Line
Tel: 0800 882200
Minicom: 0800 243355
Website: www.dwp.gov.uk
N. Ireland: 0800 220674

Government agency giving information and advice on
sickness and disability benefits for people with
disabilities and their carers.

British Lung Foundation
73–75 Goswell Road
London EC1V 7ER
Helpline: 0845 850 5020
Website: www.lunguk.org

Raises funds for research into all forms of lung disease.
Offers information leaflets and has a series of self-help
groups around the country, The Breathe Easy Club,
largely run by patients.

Midlands Asthma and Allergy Research Association (MAARA)
No. 1 Mill, The Wharf, Shardlow

Derby DE72 2GH
Tel: 01332 799600
Website: www.maara.org

A research and support association offering advice and information for people with asthma and allergies, their families as well as health professionals.

National Institute for Health and Clinical Excellence (NICE)

MidCity Place, 71 High Holborn
London WC1V 6NA
Tel: 0845 003 7780
Website: www.nice.org.uk

Provides national guidance on the promotion of good health and the prevention and treatment of ill-health. Patient information leaflets are available for each piece of guidance issued.

National Respiratory Training Centre

The Athenaeum, 10 Church Street
Warwick CV34 4AB
Tel: 01926 493313
Website: www.nrtc.org.uk

Aims to provide a consistent, comprehensive and innovative approach to professional health training in the fields of allergic conditions, respiratory health, cardiovascular disease and diabetes.

NHS Direct

Tel: 0845 4647 (24 hours, 365 days a year)
Website: www.nhsdirect.nhs.uk

Offers confidential health-care advice, information and referral service. A good first port of call for any health advice.

NHS Smoking Helpline

Freephone: 0800 169 0169 (7am–11pm, 365 days a year)
Website: www.givingupsmoking.co.uk
Pregnancy smoking helpline: 0800 169 9169
(12 noon–9pm, 365 days a year)

Have advice, help and encouragement on giving up smoking. Specialist advisers available to offer ongoing support to those who genuinely are trying to give up smoking. Can refer to local branches.

Quit (Smoking Quitlines)

211 Old Street
London EC1V 9NR
Tel: 020 7251 1551
Helpline: 0800 002200 (9am–9pm, 365 days a year)
Website: www.quit.org.uk
Scotland: 0800 848484
Wales: 0800 169 0169 (NHS)

Offers individual advice on giving up smoking in English and Asian languages. Talks to schools on smoking and pregnancy and can refer to local support groups. Runs training courses for professionals.

Useful websites
Asthma and Allergy Information and Research
www.users.globalnet.co.uk/~aair
Medical home page of MAARA.

BBC
www.bbc.co.uk/health
A helpful website: easy to navigate and offers lots of useful advice and information. Also contains links to other related topics.

Patient UK
www.patient.co.uk
Patient care website.

The internet as a source of further information

After reading this book, you may feel that you would like further information on the subject. The internet is of course an excellent place to look and there are many websites with useful information about medical disorders, related charities and support groups.

For those who do not have a computer at home some bars and cafes offer facilities for accessing the internet. These are listed in the *Yellow Pages* under 'Internet Bars and Cafes' and 'Internet Providers'. Your local library offers a similar facility and has staff to help you find the information that you need.

It should always be remembered, however, that the internet is unregulated and anyone is free to set up a website and add information to it. Many websites offer impartial advice and information that has been compiled and checked by qualified medical professionals. Some, on the other hand, are run by commercial organisations with the purpose of promoting their own products. Others still are run by pressure groups, some of which will provide carefully assessed and accurate information whereas others may be suggesting medications or treatments that are not supported by the medical and scientific community.

Unless you know the address of the website you want to visit – for example, www.familydoctor.co.uk – you may find the following guidelines useful when searching the internet for information.

Search engines and other searchable sites

Google (www.google.co.uk) is the most popular search engine used in the UK, followed by Yahoo! (http://uk.yahoo.com) and MSN (www.msn.co.uk). Also popular are the search engines provided by Internet Service Providers such as Tiscali and other sites such as the BBC site (www.bbc.co.uk).

In addition to the search engines that index the whole web, there are also medical sites with search facilities, which act almost like mini-search engines, but cover only medical topics or even a particular area of medicine. Again, it is wise to look at who is responsible for compiling the information offered to ensure that it is impartial and medically accurate. The NHS Direct site (www.nhsdirect.nhs.uk) is an example of a searchable medical site.

Links to many British medical charities can be found at the Association of Medical Research Charities' website (www.amrc.org.uk) and at Charity Choice (www.charitychoice.co.uk).

Search phrases

Be specific when entering a search phrase. Searching for information on 'cancer' will return results for many different types of cancer as well as on cancer in general. You may even find sites offering astrological information. More useful results will be returned by using search phrases such as 'lung cancer' and 'treatments for lung cancer'. Both Google and Yahoo! offer an advanced search option that includes the ability to search for the exact phrase; enclosing the search phrase in quotes, that is, 'treatments for lung cancer', will have the same effect. Limiting a search to an exact phrase reduces the number of results returned but it is best to refine a search to an exact match only if you are not getting useful results with a normal search. Adding 'UK' to your search term will bring up mainly British sites, so a good phrase might be 'lung cancer' UK (don't include UK within the quotes).

Always remember the internet is international and unregulated. It holds a wealth of valuable information but individual sites may be biased, out of date or just plain wrong. Family Doctor Publications accepts no responsibility for the content of links published in this series.

Index

Your pages

We have included the following pages because they may help you manage your illness or condition and its treatment.

Before an appointment with a health professional, it can be useful to write down a short list of questions of things that you do not understand, so that you can make sure that you do not forget anything.

Some of the sections may not be relevant to your circumstances.

We are always pleased to receive constructive criticism or suggestions about how to improve the books. You can contact us at:

Email: familydoctor@btinternet.com
Letter: Family Doctor Publications
          PO Box 4664
          Poole
          BH15 1NN

Thank you

Health-care contact details

Name:

Job title:

Place of work:

Tel:

Name:

Job title:

Place of work:

Tel:

Name:

Job title:

Place of work:

Tel:

Name:

Job title:

Place of work:

Tel:

Significant past health events – illnesses/operations/investigations/treatments

Event	Month	Year	Age (at time)

Appointments for health care

Name:

Place:

Date:

Time:

Tel:

Name:

Place:

Date:

Time:

Tel:

Name:

Place:

Date:

Time:

Tel:

Name:

Place:

Date:

Time:

Tel:

Appointments for health care

Name:

Place:

Date:

Time:

Tel:

Name:

Place:

Date:

Time:

Tel:

Name:

Place:

Date:

Time:

Tel:

Name:

Place:

Date:

Time:

Tel:

Current medication(s) prescribed by your doctor

Medicine name:

Purpose:

Frequency & dose:

Start date:

End date:

Medicine name:

Purpose:

Frequency & dose:

Start date:

End date:

Medicine name:

Purpose:

Frequency & dose:

Start date:

End date:

Medicine name:

Purpose:

Frequency & dose:

Start date:

End date:

Other medicines/supplements you are taking, not prescribed by your doctor

Medicine/treatment:

Purpose:

Frequency & dose:

Start date:

End date:

Medicine/treatment:

Purpose:

Frequency & dose:

Start date:

End date:

Medicine/treatment:

Purpose:

Frequency & dose:

Start date:

End date:

Medicine/treatment:

Purpose:

Frequency & dose:

Start date:

End date:

Questions to ask at appointments
(Note: do bear in mind that doctors work under great time pressure, so long lists may not be helpful for either of you)